Poison, detection, and
the Victorian imagination

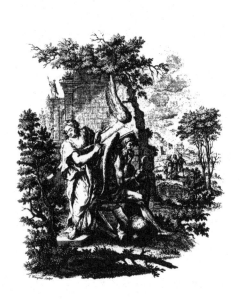

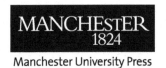
MANCHESTER
1824

Manchester University Press

ENCOUNTERS   cultural histories

Series editors:
Roger Cooter
Harriet Ritvo
Carolyn Steedman
Bertrand Taithe

Over the past few decades cultural history has become the discipline of encounters. Beyond the issues raised by the 'linguistic turn', the work of theorists such as Norbert Elias, Pierre Bourdieu, Michel Foucault or Jacques Derrida has contributed to the emergence of cultural history as a forum for bold and creative exchange. This series proposes to place encounters – human, intellectual and disciplinary – at the heart of historical thinking. *Encounters* will include short, innovative and theoretically informed books from all fields of history. The series will provide an arena for exploring new and reassembled historical subjects, stimulating perceptions and re-perceptions of the past, and methodological challenges and innovations; it will publish at history's cutting edge. The *Encounters* series will demonstrate that history is the hidden narrative of modernity.

Poison, detection, and the Victorian imagination

IAN BURNEY

Manchester University Press

Manchester and New York

Distributed exclusively in the USA by Palgrave

Published by Manchester University Press
Oxford Road, Manchester M13 9NR, UK
and Room 400, 175 Fifth Avenue, New York, NY 10010, USA
www.manchesteruniversitypress.co.uk

Distributed in the United States exclusively by
Palgrave Macmillan, 175 Fifth Avenue,
New York, NY 10010, USA

Distributed in Canada exclusively by
UBC Press, University of British Columbia, 2029 West Mall,
Vancouver, BC, Canada V6T 1Z2

British Library Cataloguing-in-Publication Data is available

Library of Congress Cataloging-in-Publication Data is available

ISBN 978 0 7190 8778 3 paperback

First published by Manchester University Press in hardback 2006

This paperback edition first published 2012

The publisher has no responsibility for the persistence or accuracy of URLs for any external or third-party internet websites referred to in this book, and does not guarantee that any content on such websites is, or will remain, accurate or appropriate.

Printed by Lightning Source

Contents

Plates

Acknowledgements

I began working on this book during my final year at the Michigan Society of Fellows, and then took it to Warwick's Centre for Social History, where I spent eighteen months as a Wellcome Research Fellow. I would like to thank colleagues and staff at both these institutions for providing me with supportive environments within which to pursue my research. Most of the research and writing has been conducted since my arrival at the University of Manchester's Centre for the History of Science, Technology and Medicine and its associated Wellcome Unit for the History of Medicine, and I have benefited greatly from the institutional and intellectual resources at my disposal here. I owe a special debt of gratitude to my Centre colleagues past and present, especially Roberta Bivins, Vladimir Jankovic, Jay Kennedy, Gill Mawson, Neil Pemberton, John Pickstone, and Mick Worboys, who have read and commented on significant portions of the manuscript. I have also enjoyed the help and encouragement of friends from the wider University community, Bob di Napoli, Conrad Leyser, and Bertrand Taithe, and the John Rylands University Library staff, especially Joanne Crane and Alyson Offiler. José Bertomeu-Sánchez and Bettina Wahrig have shared their considerable expertise on nineteenth-century toxicology with me, while Mario Biagioli, Tom Green, Chris Lawrence, Joan Scott, James Vernon, and Dror Wahrman offered their advice and critical insight throughout. The Wellcome Trust has funded my research over the life of this project, and I gratefully acknowledge its generosity.

A version of chapter 3 appeared in 'Languages of the lab: toxicological testing and medico-legal proof', in *Studies in history and philosophy of science*, 33:2, 2002, 289–314, and is reproduced here by permission of Elsevier Ltd.; portions of chapter 4 appear in 'A poisoning of no substance: the trials of medico-legal proof in mid-Victorian England', in the *Journal of British studies* 38:1 (January 1999), 59–92, and is reproduced here by permission of the University of Chicago Press.

Rachel, Cailin, and Rohin have put up with having a husband and father whose research topic might give others less loving and trusting pause for thought. I will try to find something more cheerful to write about next time. I dedicate this book to my parents, who support me in all that I do.

To my parents

Introduction

'I am innocent of poisoning Cook by strychnine'. With these words William Palmer went to the scaffold, convicted of having perpetrated the very crime he denied to the last.[1] His twelve-day trial in May 1856, described by the *Law times* as 'the longest, greatest, gravest and most important criminal trial of the nineteenth century', ended just as it had begun – with a question hanging over the central contention against him.[2] By its close, most interested observers had become convinced of his utter villainy: a gambler, a forger, an adulterer, and a serial poisoner who perverted his standing as a licensed medical practitioner to further his murderous ends, Palmer's fate provoked little in the way of sympathy. Yet his enigmatic conduct in the days and hours leading to his execution provoked widely articulated concerns, precisely because it seemed to mirror and reinforce the equally enigmatic features of his case. Palmer had been convicted of murdering his friend and gambling associate John Parsons Cook along 'scientific' lines, secretly employing carefully calibrated, minute doses of strychnine to poison without a trace. This had resulted in a gap at the centre of the case against him: although strychnine was named as the poison that had killed Cook, none was detected in his body.

Lingering doubts about the accuracy of the scientific evidence against him, then, was what made Palmer's actions as he awaited execution a focal point for the anxiety built up over the course of the trial, and gave him a huge stage on which to perform his part. Crowds estimated as high as 50,000 in number gathered in Stafford to witness his execution, and newspapers from all over the country sent representatives to record Palmer's final hours. Their reports typically focused on a couple of key themes. First, the general air of disciplined calmness displayed by the prisoner. He ate and slept well, conversed easily with prison officials, and walked to the scaffold with 'a jaunty air and tripping gait'. Even in death he appeared to exercise self-control, *The Times* correspondent noting that a handkerchief that he had taken with him to the scaffold 'still remained tightly clenched when the body was cut down'.[3]

This calm and purposive display reinforced the effect of the second core feature of the press reports – their account of Palmer's response to official efforts at eliciting a confession. 'From the time of his sentence to the very moment when he ascended the scaffold', one correspondent observed, 'Palmer was persuaded, entreated, implored day by day, almost hour by hour, to confess his crimes, not to God, but to man'.[4] Official hopes for a confession were shared by the multitude assembled at the gallows, who, reports noted, observed an 'intense silence' during the whole of the execution spectacle.[5] An air of expectant attention is of course a generic feature of the spectacle of crime and punishment – scaffold speeches being traditional opportunities for achieving closure on a case. But reports claimed to detect what one commentator described as 'an excessive anxiety' for a confessional resolution, an anxiety that seemed to stem from the unresolved elements of the trial.[6]

In this uneasy climate, the very act of looking to Palmer to corroborate the case against him seemed to many a counter-productive exercise. 'It is to be regretted that endeavours were made to extort confession, for the assumption should always be that the crime has been proved beyond a doubt by the process of law', the *Examiner* declared. 'We are convinced that no circumstance has had half the influence in creating doubt of Palmer's guilt', the *Journal of mental science* ventured, 'as the assiduous solicitation, we may almost say persecution, for confession, to which he has been exposed'.[7] Observers surely would not have been so critical of such official 'persecution' had the result been different – had Palmer not used the opportunity to stoke the embers of controversy. With his careful statement, Palmer offered instead of closure a riddle, neither directly denying his guilt nor ratifying the grounds upon which his conviction rested. Participants and commentators reacted strongly to Palmer's parting salvo, many sharing the unconcealed exasperation of the prison governor when he exhorted Palmer to stop 'quibbling'. 'Are you guilty of the murder?' he reportedly demanded, adding 'It is of very little importance how the deed was done'.[8]

This book is predicated on the proposition that the governor was wrong – that it *did* matter how the deed was done. It certainly mattered in the limited instance of Palmer's trial, as commentators seized upon the possible implications embedded in his ambiguous declaration. 'It will be seen that the convict contented himself with denying that Cook was poisoned by strychnine, and that no direct answer was ever given by him

to the question whether he murdered him by other means', *The Times*
observed. 'Should there be any foundation for the suggestion that the
death was caused by other means', it concluded gravely, 'it would tend still
further to complicate this most extraordinary case'.[9] This suggestion –
that Palmer's declaration might serve as a legitimate, if unwelcome, basis
for re-opening the scientific debates so openly and contentiously aired in
the courtroom, also featured in medical and scientific comment on his
execution. The *Association medical journal* concluded its scaffold report
on a note of strikingly unconcealed disappointment:

> The hope that Palmer in his last moments would make such a confession as
> would clear up once and for ever the doubts that still remain in the minds
> of many persons as to his guilt, has been disappointed; and his last words
> will, we fear, only tend to strengthen the opinion of those who denied that
> Mr. Cook died from the effects of strychnine. The few words that the
> wretched criminal uttered before proceeding to the scaffold, instead of
> clearing up the difficulties which have beset the minds of many medical
> men, will only tend to still further perplex them.[10]

As an example of considered medical reflection, the *Journal*'s editorial is
remarkable. Its recourse to the convention of dying declarations as a
necessary supplement to a form of evidence that, as a medical journal, it
purported to represent, speaks volumes about the sense of unresolved-
ness that persisted after the trial, and not merely amongst a credulous
public. Medical men had sought confirmation in the scaffold's traditional
promise of clarity and truth, and had been disappointed, even perplexed,
by what it appeared to have told them.[11]

The prison governor was wrong in a larger sense as well. Beyond the
particularities of the Palmer case, determining the means used by poisoners to accomplish their ends was of vital importance in responses to
criminal poisoning in Victorian Britain. Through an analysis of criminal
poisoning and the social, cultural, legal and scientific responses it elicited,
this book seeks to show how and why this was so.[12]

The poison discussed in the coming pages is limited to that used (or
thought to be used) for criminal purposes, 'detection' in turn referring to
toxicology and the ancillary medico-legal knowledges that might be
brought to bear on a case of suspected criminal poisoning. Focusing on
this dimension to the exclusion of other, broader possibilities (environmental or aetiological conceptions of poison, for example) enables an
exploration, in the first instance, of a richly textured historical example of
the application of medical and scientific expertise to matters of criminal
law. Yet the crime of poisoning in Victorian Britain leads into areas that

exceed the expected limits of medico-legal expertise, ones in which different imaginations – historical, literary, legal and scientific – converge to position poison as an object of fascination, and as an object of knowledge.

The specifics of this statement are better left to the arguments laid out in the chapters to come. However, the following observation might be of use as an indicator of the path ahead: poison, expert detection, and the imagination each intersect in suggestive ways with the concept of absence. Definitions of imagination (whether as a substantive – a faculty of the mind – or an action of this faculty) commonly specify its relationship to a world of absent things, the *Oxford English Dictionary*'s primary entry for 'imagination' characterizing it as 'the action of imagining, or forming a mental concept of what is not actually present to the senses'.[13] In general usage, this quality of calling into being something not immediately perceptible often carries pejorative overtones, a suggestion that the concept formed by the imagination is a mere fantasy, the product of an ill-disciplined mind.[14] But this is not a necessary connotation, the relationship between the imaginative and the real being capable of greater complexity than that of straightforward opposition. Indeed, the epistemological status of the imagination's capacity to call the impalpable into being has been a matter of running debate since classical times, regarded (often simultaneously) as a source of creative power and of error. In enabling understanding beyond immediate sense impulse, the imagination is accorded an indispensable role in generating knowledge of the world. Yet to the extent that it is driven by the desire to recall or conjure that which is absent, it carries within it the seeds of delusion, sin or madness.[15]

This tension between the imagination as an asset and a liability featured prominently in late eighteenth- and early nineteenth-century discussions about the basis of human cognition, as critics of a strict empiricist and associationist epistemology sought out routes to reliable knowledge lying beyond the realm of immediate sense perception.[16] This was a subject with profound resonances in contemporary accounts of science. As Jonathan Smith has argued, nineteenth-century scientists, although in important respects heirs to the empiricist tradition, did not regard the imagination as wholly inimical to objective knowledge – instead seeing it as an often necessary component of its production.[17]

Smith assembles a wide range of commentators who conceived of the relationship as one of dynamic tension: while agreeing that the imagination required disciplining in order to be turned to scientific use, they equally rejected a crude version of Baconian fact-gathering devoid of the imagination. The acclaimed early nineteenth-century chemist Humphry Davy, although insisting that scientific knowledge should be sought not in the 'fancies of men, but in the visible and tangible external world', also commended the imagination as 'a noble instrument of discovery'.[18] Justus Liebig, another of the century's chemical luminaries, expressed a similar split between the creative and dangerous facets of the imagination. An implacable foe of what he considered the ungrounded delusions of German *Naturphilosophie*, Liebig at the same time embraced the scientific imagination, observing that 'the mental faculty which constitutes the poet and the artist is the same as that whence discoveries and progress in science spring'. As Smith notes, this celebration of the disciplined but creative mind of science found a ready echo amongst social commentators, with G. H. Lewes – journalist, critic and expositor of both Goethe and Comte – declaring that science 'mounts on the wings of Imagination into regions of the invisible and impalpable'.[19]

The world of Victorian criminal poisoning constituted an exemplary region of the invisible and impalpable. Conceived as an act committed in the absence of direct and visible contact between perpetrator and victim, poisoning appeared as a form of violence that operated beneath the threshold of perception. Its material effects on the body, moreover, were construed as evanescent, especially in the hands of a skilled practitioner. It was a crime that thus has to be traced out from evidence of the unseen. In this sense, poison operated inextricably at the level of the imagination as defined and debated by contemporaries. Not actually present to the senses in its substantive form, it required a faculty of mind capable of forming a concept of things not present. The poison 'detective', consequently, was someone for whom an imagination could prove an asset – if one that required vigilance and restraint.

If the detection of things not immediately present to the senses was the hallmark of poison detection, it should also be noted that the presence/absence fault-line is also central to a more limited legal conception of expert testimony. In its original and commonly applied usage, 'expert' derives from the Latin 'to try', and refers to experience in and of something, often connected with a particular skill- and knowledge-set derived from this experience. Another, more esoteric, etymological root links expert to '*expert-em*', translated as 'having no part in'. In this sense, expert can be defined as 'destitute or devoid of, free from', and, in the context of Anglo-American legal theory, this secondary definition connects with the more common one in a suggestive way. Expert evidence as a special category, in this tradition, is a product of the late eighteenth century, when restrictions on the admissibility of testimony derived from both indirect observation or knowledge and opinion were applied to witnesses in general. Expert witnesses were recognized exceptions to these exclusionary rules – an expert was someone who, as Thomas Starkie observed, was allowed to give an opinion on matters before the court which were established by the evidence of others, 'and without being personally acquainted with the facts'.[20]

It is not surprising then, that from a popular, scientific, and legal standpoint, it was the poison detective – the toxicologist – who emerged as the leading representative of the growing field of nineteenth-century medico-legal expertise. The toxicologist acted as a mediator between the insensible and the sensible, his task to demonstrate the presence of things not evident to others. He thus occupied the space of creative tension between different regions of fact and imagination. His standing as a model of modern scientific expertise owed much to the hold that poison exercised on the imagination of the Victorian public. It was, as one medico-legal author observed, his power to neutralize poison's widely attributed intangibility that 'cause[s] the vulgar to marvel at the mysterious power by which an atom of arsenic mingled amidst a mass of confused ingesta can still be detected'.[21] But while public acclaim for his proofs might be derived from this sense of mysterious power, his actions as a matter of science were properly grounded in hard, material fact. He was no mere magician. And yet, toxicology in practice, much like the broader Victorian discourse on poison, was haunted by the difficulties of getting hold of and providing a stable representation of this illusive agent of crime. Poison detection called on creative acts of perception on the part of its experts: of analytical results that required a degree of imagination to secure their standing as matters of fact.

It is this vision of poison – the collective product of the Victorian public, legal and scientific imagination – that will be pursued in what follows. Chapter 1 explores how contemporary observers located criminal poisoning within a multi-layered network of historical and cultural references. Within this network of references, poison emerged as a way of reflecting on the nature of mid-nineteenth century 'civilization' – what it had wrought, what challenged it, and what could be marshalled to defend it. Chapter 2 focuses on the painstaking attempts to construct a 'modern' conceptual and legislative framework for containing the threat posed by criminal poisoning. In these efforts, proponents of toxicology engaged with the cultural meanings associated with modern poisoning, seeking to rewrite poison's past and present in a way that would secure for science a recognized role in combating its dangers. Chapter 3 moves from efforts to delineate the terms of scientific engagement with modern poison to an analysis of how toxicological work was undertaken and represented. The two critical sites for this analysis are the toxicological laboratory on the one hand, and the criminal courtroom on the other. In their labs, toxicologists wrestled with a complex phenomenology of detection, attempting to translate often ambiguous smells, taste, and colours (phenomena which they themselves recognized as speaking to the imagination of the observer) into definitive and agreed-upon indications of poison. In the courtroom, their labours were multiplied: here they were constrained to negotiate with a public steeped in poison lore, and with an adversarial legal process which drew on this imaginative register to 'test' their expert testimony.

These chapters, then, develop an analysis of the different 'cultures' of poison as distinct but mutually constituting elements. Toxicology's standing as the pre-eminent representative of Victorian medico-legal expertise, they demonstrate, cannot be understood without reference to the broader anxieties engendered by criminal poisoning. Toxicology, furthermore, was central to these concerns, as Victorians were exposed to and cognizant of its claims and techniques, and critically assessed its capacity to meet its objectives. Here poisoning trials served as anchoring points, at once opportunities for illustrating the significance of poisoning in concrete instances, and stages for the display of the capacities and limits of scientific expertise. The final two chapters are tethered to the most notorious of these anchoring points – the case of William Palmer. In motive and means, Palmer's was the quintessential 'crime of civilization', and chapter 4 shows how his case was enmeshed with a core set of concerns about the social and cultural underpinnings of a self-consciously 'modern' Britain. The case also served to focus attention on the civilized response to criminal poisoning, revealing a gap between public and scientific evidentiary expectations, and suggesting that the science of poison detection was not exempt from the problems it was called upon to resolve. Chapter 5 examines toxicology in the aftermath of the Palmer trial, showing how the tensions it highlighted within the imaginative landscape of Victorian poisoning led to an implosion of the toxicological project. The epic framing of toxicology's struggles with poison and the poisoner yielded to two (seemingly contradictory) revisions: on the one hand, to a more modest, less individually heroic role for the poison hunter, a vision of expertise as the collective application of consensually developed knowledge; and, on the other, to a literary reworking of the constitutive elements of toxicology's quest for mastery, a transposed re-articulation of the fraught relationship between poison, detection, and the Victorian imagination.

Notes

1 Although not Palmer's last reported words, this was the statement that most press reports represented as his final declaration. The newspaper coverage of Palmer's trial and execution has been analysed by Thomas Boyle, *Black swine in the sewers of Hampstead: beneath the surface of Victorian sensationalism* (London: Penguin, 1989), chs 8–9, and, for the contemporary medical press, by Michael Harris, 'Social diseases? crime and medicine in the Victorian press', in W. F. Bynum, Stephen Lock and Roy Porter (eds), *Medical journals and medical knowledge* (London: Routledge, 1992), pp. 108–25.

2 'The great trial', *Law times* 7 (1856), p. 110.

3 'The Rugeley poisonings. The execution of Palmer', *The Times* (16 June 1856), p. 9.

4 'The trial and execution of William Palmer', *Journal of mental science* 2 (1856), p. 513.

5 *Lloyd's weekly newspaper* (15 June 1856), p. 12.

6 'Palmer's end', *Examiner* (21 June 1856), p. 386.

7 *Ibid.*; *Journal of mental science*, p. 514.

8 'Our civilization. Execution of William Palmer', *Leader* (21 June 1856), pp. 582–3, p. 582.

9 'The Rugeley poisonings. The execution of Palmer', *The Times* (16 June 1856), p. 9.

10 'The last moments of Palmer', *Association medical journal* 4 (n.s.) (1856), pp. 521–2, p. 521.

11 Those *AMJ* readers of a phrenological bent might have taken heart at the results of the final interrogation to which Palmer was submitted on his day of execution. An examination of his skull found that 'it was physically impossible for him ever to have been a good man', revealing one particular feature that would mark him out as an exemplary poisoner: in the middle region of his skull, phrenologists found the formation corresponding to the trait of secretiveness 'remarkably prominent'. 'Execution of William Palmer', *Leader* (21 June 1856), p. 583. Palmer's mastery of poisoning – that most secret of crimes – was written on his body.

12 In recent years, several scholars have considered the topic of Victorian criminal poisoning. Katherine Watson's *Poisoned lives: English poisoners and their victims* (London and New York: London and Hambeldon, 2004) approaches the topic from a social historical perspective; George Robb, 'Circe in crinoline: domestic poisonings in Victorian England', *Journal of family history*, 22:2

(1997), pp. 176–90, and Judith Knelman, *Twisting in the wind: the murderess and the English press* (Toronto, Buffalo and London: University of Toronto Press, 1998), emphasize the gendered dimension of criminal poisoning; my focus on the intersection of public, legal and scientific cultures of poison is shared by Mark Essig's 'Science and sensation: poison murder and forensic medicine in nineteenth-century America', Ph.D. dissertation, Cornell University, 2000.

13 This is a definition endorsed by contemporary commentators: the lexicologist Samuel Johnson (for whom the imagination played a crucial role in the rise of a 'civilized' sensibility), conceived it as primarily 'the power of representing things absent', while John Stuart Mill (in his critique of utilitarianism's prosaic tendencies), endorsed the view of 'the best writers of the present day' that the imagination was 'that which enables us, by a voluntary effort, to conceive the absent as if it were present'. Samuel Johnson, *Dictionary of the English language*, cited in James Engell, *The creative imagination: Enlightenment to Romanticism* (Cambridge MA and London: Harvard University Press, 1981), p. 57; John Stuart Mill, *Essay on Bentham and Coleridge*, cited in John Whale, *The imagination under pressure, 1789–1832* (Cambridge: Cambridge University Press, 2000), p. 181. Johnson's eighteenth-century definition is retained in its many re-editions published in the first half of the nineteenth century.

14 The *OED* notes that the term is used 'often with implication that the conception does not correspond to the reality of things'.

15 For an introduction to classical concepts of the imagination, see J. M. Cocking, *Imagination: a study in the history of ideas* (London: Routledge, 1991).

16 This critique is most commonly associated with – though by no means limited to – Romantic accounts of cognition. For guides to this topic, see, in addition to Engell's *Creative imagination*, and Whale's *Imagination under pressure*, M. H. Abrams's classic *The mirror and the lamp: Romantic theory and the critical tradition* (London, Oxford and New York: Oxford University Press, 1953).

17 Jonathan Smith, *Fact and feeling: Baconian science and the nineteenth-century literary imagination* (Madison and London: University of Wisconsin Press, 1994). The following paragraph is indebted to Smith's analysis, especially chs 1–2. For a different account of the relationship between science and the imagination which, though also recognizing the productive role attributed to the imagination, stresses the increasing attempts to marginalize it as a threat to the emergent ideals of objectivity in nineteenth-century science, see Lorraine Daston, 'Fear and loathing of the imagination in science', *Daedalus* 127:1 (1998), pp. 73–93.

18 Humphry Davy, cited in Smith, *Fact and feeling*, pp. 15, 82. Davy, of course, was himself an exemplary instance of the early nineteenth-century overlap of Romanticism and science, his chemistry celebrated by Coleridge as a natural-

ized version of the imagination's capacity to move beyond the level of mere sense. For more on this, see Trevor Levere, *Poetry realized in nature: Samuel Taylor Coleridge and early nineteenth-century science* (Cambridge: Cambridge University Press, 1981), especially ch. 1 and 6.

19 Justus Liebig, 'Lord Bacon as natural philosopher' (1863); G. H. Lewes, *The foundations of a creed* (1874–75), cited in Smith, *Fact and feeling*, pp. 35–6. As Smith notes, the physicist John Tyndall, who along with Huxley represented the apex of scientific materialism, nevertheless insisted that scientists must use imagination in order to transcend the limits of merely present. Tyndall's influential address on 'Scientific use of the imagination', in Smith's account, itself became incorporated as a catchphrase for what was lacking in crude versions of Baconianism.

20 Thomas Starkie, *Practical treatise on the law of evidence*, 2 vols, 2nd edn (London: J. and W. T. Clarke, 1833), 1, p. 154. As Thomas Peake explained in 1801, it was the expert's command of a field of scientific knowledge that enabled him to act in this capacity: 'Though witnesses can in general speak only as to facts, yet in questions of science, persons versed in the subject, may deliver their opinions upon oath, on the case proved by the other witnesses'. Peake illustrates this with the case of a physician who, on the basis of evidence provided by other witnesses, was permitted to testify to the effects and likely consequences of a disease, despite the fact that he 'has not seen the particular patient' (Peake, cited in Stephan Landsman, 'One-hundred years of rectitude: medical witnesses at the Old Bailey, 1717–1817', *Law and history review* 16:3 (1998), pp. 445–94, p. 493). There is a growing literature on the legal application of scientific expertise. For more on the development of the concept and practice of expert evidence in the English context, see, in addition to Landsman, Tal Golan, 'The history of scientific expert testimony in the English courtroom', *Science in context* 12:1 (1999), pp. 7–32 and Tal Golan, *Laws of men and laws of nature: the history of scientific expert testimony in England and America* (Cambridge MA and London: Harvard University Press, 2004). For the problematic application of medico-legal expertise to another realm of the unseen – insanity cases – see Roger Smith, *Trial by medicine: insanity and responsibility in Victorian trials* (Edinburgh: Edinburgh University Press, 1981), and Joel Eigen, *Witnessing insanity: madness and mad-doctors in the English court* (London and New Haven: Yale University Press, 1995).

21 T. R. Beck, cited in W. M. Best, *A treatise on the principles of evidence and practice as to proofs in courts of common law; with elementary rules for conducting the examination and cross-examination of witnesses* (London: S. Sweet, 1849), p. 388.

1

Poison and the Victorian imagination

Thomas de Quincey, in his 1827 essay 'On Murder, considered as one of the fine arts', adopted the role of connoisseur of this most peculiar of art forms. Selecting exemplary instances from the recent annals of British crime, de Quincey's murder critic professed a clear preference for shedders of blood, condemning less sanguinary methods in forthright terms: 'Fie on these dealers in poison, say I: can they not keep to the old honest way of cutting throats, without introducing such abominable innovations from Italy?'[1]

De Quincey, himself no stranger to the allure of noxious substances, surely did not intend to have his essay taken at face value. Yet within three decades commentators were doing just that, professing a profound lack of comprehension of de Quincey's aesthetic sensibility. If one were to discuss murder as a fine art, they argued, surely so discerning an observer would not single out crude physical assault. He would instead focus on what mid-nineteenth century commentators insisted was the archetypal instrument of modern violence. Looking back on de Quincey's essay, an 1859 editorial in the progressive weekly, *Leader,* declared that he had failed to recognize the delights of 'a good poisoning case', in which the criminal 'moves through circumstances of mystery, . . . and keeps brains puzzling, and hearts throbbing, and betting books going, until the verdict is given'. A *Times* editorial in the following year agreed, confessing that it had 'always been surprised' at de Quincey's analysis: 'The poetry of homicide', it declared, 'belongs in a special degree to poisoning'.[2]

A decade later, the cultural critic Leslie Stephen penned an updated analysis of the homicidal arts, which appeared as 'The decay of murder' in a *Cornhill magazine* essay signed by 'A cynic'. In this revisitation of de Quincey, Stephen's cynic comments on those who professed to mourn the passing of an era of 'heroic' murder. According to this view, de Quincey's cut-throat was symptomatic of a more direct era of 'picturesque' individuality and authentic action. Yet for Stephen's cynic, this lament had less to do with homicide itself, than with the uneasy recognition of a more fundamental social shift constitutive of the modern world: 'We are fallen', he complains, 'upon the days of petty passions and commonplace characters. Our modern heroes are marked by an absence of the ancient energy. One man is more and more like his neighbour. The object of our costume is no longer to set off the personal advantages which our figures may possess, but to enable them to escape all notice in a crowd'.[3]

The decline of violent crime, in this analysis, is the product of civilized refinement, though not necessarily a measure of progress: 'That we do not commit great crimes is owing less to any positive advance in virtue than to a general desire to conform to the average standard'. The 'enervating polish of civilization', Stephen concluded, has 'insidiously transform[ed] us into a very dull, highly respectable, and intensely monotonous collection of insignificant units'.[4]

Taken together, these re-readings of de Quincey delineate a modern aesthetics of criminal violence, in which bold physicality had been displaced by a more insidious form of subterranean (or sub-cutaneous) violation. In the interval between de Quincey and Stephen, criminal poisoning had come to be recognized as a distinctly modern phenomenon. It was, as the *Illustrated times* declared in 1856, at once the 'crime of the age', and 'the crime of civilization'.[5] The aim of this chapter is to examine the interlocking elements out of which Victorian commentators constructed an understanding of poisoning as, in important respects, a specifically modern concern. This identification of poisoning as modern relied upon a conceptual framework forged from an inherited (and nurtured) politico-historical narrative; a contemporary examination of the nature of 'civilization'; and the cultural, historical, and material meanings attributable to poison as an instrument of crime. This 'public' discourse on poison reached out to broader contemporary concerns, stimulating reflection on the attainments and shortcomings of modern society.

In singling out secret poisoning as 'the crime of civilization', the *Illustrated times* and others like it were at once providing a diagnosis of contemporary society, and a comparison with specific historical antecedents. In such analyses, poison figured as a self-consciously historicized phenomenon, by means of which the peculiarities of the modern world came into sharp relief. Indeed, the journal announced that it had adapted its term 'crime of the age' from one of the leading political and historical commentators of the day, Thomas Babington Macaulay. The phrase, appropriately enough, was drawn from Macaulay's essay analysing

Machiavelli's legacy for a modern conception of politics. Although a term of vilification in the nineteenth-century political lexicon, 'Machiavellianism', Macaulay observed, had been in its own time a legitimate tool of political art. This was due to the state of civilization to which Machiavelli's Italy had risen (or fallen), where duplicity was not considered a vice, but an acceptable means to an end. For the Renaissance statesman, Macaulay explained, 'to do an injury openly is . . . as wicked as to do it secretly, and far less profitable. With him the most honourable means are – the surest, the speediest, and the darkest . . . He would think it madness to declare open hostilities against a rival whom he might stab in a friendly embrace, or poison in a consecrated wafer'.[6] Macaulay's invocation of poison as a once appropriate but now unacceptable tool of political art, tapped into a rich and complex vein of associations between poison and crime familiar to his contemporaries. Poison was Italian, dangerously refined, and, in its historical incarnation, an instrument of high politics.

Italian political history, encompassing both classical Roman and Renaissance courts, served as an instructive touchstone for Victorian commentary on poison. Locating poison in space and time as 'Italian' was, of course, nothing new, as Victorian commentators were able to draw on a long line of associations transmitted through influential representational genres of past epochs. In medieval saint's lives, corrupt Italian monks might resort to the poisoned chalice to stave off externally imposed programmes of reform.[7] Poisoned bibles, portraits, and candles at work in imperial and Renaissance courts littered the Elizabethan and Jacobean stage. For the likes of Ben Jonson, Christopher Marlowe, and John Webster, such poisonous practices could serve a number of figurative purposes: as a comment on the decadent Italianate and papist English court rife with poison intrigue; and as a metaphor for social 'falseness' more generally, in which the pursuit of self-interest and greed by the manipulation of appearance threatened to undermine traditional, native values.[8] The sweeping narratives of eighteenth-century historians invoked poison as a prism through which to view the implosion of past civilizations. 'The effeminate luxury, which infected the manners of [Roman] courts and cities', Edward Gibbon remarked, 'had instilled [in them] a secret and destructive poison', while for John Millar the 'the decay of the military spirit' in the Italian city-states of the Renaissance 'was manifest from their disuse of duelling, . . . and from their substituting in place of it the more artful but cowardly practice of poisoning'.[9]

Victorians adapted this long-standing politico-historical narrative of poisoning for their own purposes. As Norman Vance has shown, the

Victorian age witnessed a flowering of interest in ancient Rome, and in the numerous histories written in the mid-nineteenth century the link between poison and imperial decline was kept alive.[10] Liddell's 1855 *History of Rome*, to take but one example, contrasts a 'republican simplicity of manners' with an imperial decay exemplified by 'wives poisoning their husbands, and . . . the discovery of secret associations of men and women where some new and licentious worship of Bacchus was introduced'.[11] Although in some sense merely re-warming a venerable trope, stories of imperial decline took on new significance in the context of a Britain in the process of fashioning its own imperial self.[12]

Poison could serve other contemporary political projects, that of constructing a history of Whig progressivism, for example. For Macaulay, the corrupt, poison-drenched Stuart courts provided a narrative anchor on which to secure an account of the triumph of reason and morality. James I, Macaulay starkly asserted, was the first English monarch for whom the nation felt active contempt. The reason was not hard to discern: 'the perjuries, the sorceries, the poisonings' which permeated his court made James a seventeenth-century Claudius. That England as a whole did not descend into a Claudian bacchanalia was due to the solid virtues of the country, the very force that would soon arise in virtuous indignation to re-assert native (Whig) values: 'England', Macaulay rejoiced, 'was no place, the seventeenth century no time, for Sporus and Locusta'.[13] In defying the poisonous Stuart court, England had commenced a journey of re-asserting its true self, a journey which, in the Whig historical schema, had led to the virtuous present.[14]

As a historical phenomenon, then, poisoning figured within a dominant and easily recognizable account of the genealogy of a rational and virtuous civil society, a celebration of civilization in its modern English form. Yet the concept of civilization was by no means a straightforward one for Victorian commentators. For John Stuart Mill, civilization stood, on the one hand, in contrast to savagery or barbarism, characterized by forms of association that softened and curbed the brute state of nature. But, Mill asserts, 'civilized' social forms also begot what he terms 'the vices or miseries of civilization', vices that stemmed from the very same co-operative interdependence that made civilization possible. In the example most relevant to our concerns, Mill notes (following Locke) that a consequence of the marginalization of private violence attendant on civilized interdependence was the attenuation of bold action as a feature of modern sensibility, experience, and even capacity: 'The heroic', Mill observed, 'essentially consists in being ready, for a worthy object, to do

and to suffer, but especially to do, what is painful or disagreeable . . .
There has crept over the refined classes, over the whole class of gentlemen
in England, a moral effeminacy, an inaptitude for every kind of struggle'.[15]

Mill's doubts about civilized society were widely shared, as contemporaries surveyed the challenges thrown up by their imperial and industrial
present. Anxieties about the potential pitfalls of Britain's global reach
were clearly discernible even in the heyday of empire. From this perspective, the histories of classical decline spoke to a very present concern,
serving less to distinguish modern from classical civilization than to suggest possible parallels. A similar point can be made for critics of Britain's
industrial order. For Carlyle, industrial civilization was an oxymoron, the
worship of Mammon dissolving the bonds that support a virtuous community: 'We call it a Society', he raged in *Past and present*, 'and go about
professing openly the totalist separation, isolation'. For Matthew Arnold,
'depression and ennui' constituted a characteristic modern product –
symptoms 'of the disease of the most modern societies, the most
advanced civilizations'.[16]

Modern civilization also entailed a loss of legibility, the result of a physical and social mobility driven, ultimately, by the demands of the marketplace. In modern society, Mill observed, 'the individual becomes lost in
the crowd . . . An established character becomes at once more difficult to
gain, and more easily to be dispensed with'.[17] This plasticity of character,
a dark side of the civilizing process, was a theme enthusiastically
embraced in contemporary literature as well as in social and
political commentary. G. W. M. Reynolds, in his bestselling exposé of
contemporary moral disorder, *The mysteries of London*, linked civilization
to concealed, characterless criminality:

> The more civilization progresses, the more refined becomes the human
> intellect, so does human iniquity increase. It is true that heinous and
> appalling crimes are less frequent; – but every kind of social, domestic,
> political, and commercial intrigue grows more into vogue, . . . hypocrisy is
> the cloak which conceals modern acts of turpitude, as dark nights were
> trusted to for the concealment of the bloody deeds of old.[18]

It would have come as no surprise to readers of *The mysteries* that one of
its prime hypocrites, a lustful cleric, guards against exposure by means of
secret poison. Poison, in a world of anonymity, deception, and calculation, was a singularly appropriate modern tool.

It is this sense of the ambiguities of modern civilization that made
poisoning appear as its emblematic crime. Crimes of a ruder age, or of a

ruder society, were first and foremost crimes that were 'direct'. Direct in the psychology of their execution: they were spontaneous, unpremeditated, perpetrated with passion, the transparent expression of an authentic mental state. Direct, moreover, in that they used instruments of overt physicality. Bludgeons and knives depended on unmediated contact between assailant and victim and, working from the outside in, left physical traces on the body's surface. Poison could play no part in such a crude sociology of violence. In support of its claim that poison was 'the crime of civilization', the *Illustrated times* characteristically reached out to history:

> In early days, violence is the characteristic of crime, as of everything else; in latter days, craftiness or cunning. The dagger carried off the enemy in early Rome; the Emperor Claudius was poisoned . . . Indeed, as Rome became corrupt, poisoning became more and more the regular crime of the day.[19]

This widely recognized association of poison with 'refinement' depended on a set of interrelated assumptions about the way that poisoner and poison acted. Both were seen as working 'indirectly'. Poisoners, unlike the blood-drenched murderer, had a mediated relationship to their victims. They eschewed obvious, face-to-face conflict; their violence operated at a remove from the violated body; they never revealed their intentions, masking their murderous designs under precisely the opposite guise (as nurturers, or even healers). According to *The Times*, 'The man whose "feet are swift to shed blood" . . . gives signs of a savage disposition'. Contrast this with the poisoner, who 'is not a marked man. He may be a smoothfaced, plausible person, without any external symptoms of depravity, liable to no wild and furious outbursts of passion, and only "imagining mischief secretly in the deep of his heart"'.[20]

Newspaper accounts of the Victorian courtroom reinforced this idea of the inscrutable poisoner, readers typically learning that the external appearances of suspects were unreliable guides to their true actions. Catherine Foster's appearance 'pourtrays [sic] not the slightest hardihood, or anything indicating her to be a person likely to commit such a crime', while the 'good-looking and rather ladylike' Mary Ann Milner used her benign appearance to deadly advantage, luring her victims 'under the pretence of hospitality', offering poisoned cakes 'with simulated kindness'.[21] The most striking example of the enigmatic modern poisoner, judging by the editorial space devoted specially to it, was that of John Tawell. A married Buckinghamshire apothecary ostensibly devoted to 'the views, the garb, the phraseology, and the other general characteristics of the Society of Friends', in 1845 Tawell was tried and convicted of poisoning his mistress. His outward adherence (sartorial and devotional) to the ways of righteousness made his malign interior all the more compelling to his contemporaries. For the *News of the world*, Tawell presented a dangerous instance of enigmatic criminality: 'There can be no doubt that he furnishes an example of hypocrisy, a parallel for which would in vain be sought for in the criminal annals of any country'.[22] *The Times* concurred, regarding Tawell as an instructive instance of the dangers of assuming a correlation between action and appearance. 'It is felt that a man cannot assume a fair outside without some real predilection for it, and that if he is absolutely vicious, he must have lost both the power and the taste for disguise'. So long as the human capacity for true hypocrisy remained the subject of debate, it concluded, 'the case of John Tawell will occupy a prominent place in the controversy'.[23]

Poison, like the poisoner, was capable of deceitful, disguised appearances. The ideal poison was tasteless, odourless, colourless – a substance without manifest quality. As such, it could dissolve itself into the stuff of everyday life, substances that in their apparent intent were signed as benign or healthful. Its action upon the body of the victim completed the circuit of secrecy, duplicity, and interiority. It was an article of faith amongst professional and lay commentators alike that the body of the victim, in contrast to the appearance of victims of cruder violence, was illegible at the surface level: 'Nineteen-twentieths of all the poisons', the radical surgeon, politician and coroner Thomas Wakley wrote in his reformist medical journal the *Lancet*, 'leave no mark or sign of the dreadful work that has been going on internally, on the external surface of the body'. Wakley's coronial contemporary, William Baker, argued along similar lines that 'as civilisation increases, the refinement in crime keeps pace'. In 'ruder ages', Baker explained, criminality was 'of a bold and violent description, and left its traces behind, but now villainy is so refined, . . . that the murderer leaves scarcely a clue to his discovery'. Poison, in the view of Charles Dickens's *Household words*, 'seems by no means so regular a murder as a blow or a stab, which leaves marks of blood and horror'.[24] As will be demonstrated in chapter 2, this consensus on the illegibility of poison was in important respects an invention of nineteenth-century toxicology, a claim which dismissed previously held views about poison's external symptomology as relics of an 'unscientific' age. The novelty of the inscrutable poisoned body, however, did nothing to weaken its position as an article of faith.

Undetected on the outside of the body and in the appearance of the perpetrator, poison operated at a further level of 'modern' inscrutability:

that of motive. As we have already seen, historicized accounts of secret poisoning tended to associate past poisonings with high politics and 'noble' passions. As a consequence, the range of past victims, according to logic and to a selective reading of historical sources, was itself highly circumscribed. In the modern world, according to *The Times*, this had been reversed:

> There is one feature in the modern type of murders by poison which is peculiarly formidable. Unlike those of early times, they have no State reasons for their motive, and require no elaborate machinery for their execution. In these days of cheap and easy expedients crime itself has been popularized. It wears the tame and pusillanimous character so often attributed to the present generation.[25]

As Mill had predicted for civilized people generally, the modern poisoner had lost this 'heroic' cast, and was instead a mere product of a market age.

This contrast between poison's noble past and mundane present can be seen at work in one of the most widely read poison narratives of the day, Edward Bulwer Lytton's *Lucretia*. The plot of this best-selling 'romance' featured poison as the driver of a complex web of money-making schemes pursued by its principal characters. The eponymous heroine's (or anti-heroine's) name immediately recalled the exploits of Lucretia Borgia; her surname, Clavering, would have been equally resonant for a contemporary audience. Published in November 1846, only months following a notorious poisoning case centred on the Essex village of the same name, the novel's main character combined in name precisely the juxtaposition between past and present that so intrigued contemporaries (see below, pp. 26–7, 33, for details of Clavering case). Lytton, for his part, made such comparative purposes explicit. Intending to demonstrate 'the influence of Mammon upon our most secret selves, [and to] reprov[e] the impatience which is engendered by a civilization that with much of the good brings all the evils', he used Lucretia Clavering to argue that, though more pedestrian in their objects and person, modern villains were in their own terms comparable to their more obviously exalted predecessors.[26] They were capable of exhibiting 'the same attributes of character, the same alliance of the sensual and the cruel, the effeminate and unsparing, which may startle us in the imperial poisoner'. Only the superficial observer, he insisted, 'sees grandeur but in the crown or the toga'.[27] The novel itself was littered with such comparisons. Describing Lucretia's duplicitous conversation with one of her intended victims as 'a masterpiece of art', Lytton then commented: 'What pity that such craft and subtlety were wasted in our little day, and on such petty objects; under the Medici, that spirit had gone far to the shaping of history'. At another point, Lucretia herself examines her motives as a modern poisoner: 'Why should I falter in the paths which [Cesare Borgia] trod with his royal step, only because my goal is not a throne?'[28]

A developed public discourse of poison was thus a recognizable aspect of an imaginative landscape that was at once historical and historicized. As suggested by the imbrication of poison's past and present in Lytton's text, however, this discourse was not free-floating. Deeply embedded in history and culture, it was nevertheless responsive to unfolding events – most critically, to poisoning trials themselves. Accounts of Victorian poisoning trials, in this sense, drew upon a broad and interpretively flexible set of associations that were at once of descriptive and analytical use, bearing the potential to recast, as well as reinforce, the established narrative frame. Poisoning trials engaged the discourse laid out above, and elaborated it by providing contemporary, embodied referents. Indeed, the distinction between the real and imagined realms of Victorian poison is in some respects heuristic only: aspects of the above discussion have been abstracted, for the purposes of conceptualization, from specific cases which at once inflected the general discourse and gave it limiting specificity. It is now time to lay this expository fiction to one side, and to examine how the conceptual picture presented above interacted with actual Victorian poisoning cases.

Let us start with numbers. Victorian commentators clearly thought they were witnessing a 'rebirth' of the crime of poisoning. Responding to three cases brought to public attention in December, 1855, the *Saturday review* asked rhetorically: 'Is the poisoning mania, after more than two centuries of sleep, revived among us?'[29] The historical record gives us some grounds to answer with a qualified 'yes'. Historians of medieval English homicide have argued that poisoning cases, and 'stealth' modes of killing generally, were comparatively rare.[30] By the Elizabethan and Jacobean periods, however, they note the more regular presence of poisoning at criminal proceedings. F. T. Bower found a dozen criminal poisonings listed in Stowe's *Annales* between 1571 and 1598, and makes the wider claim that such texts reveal 'case after case of poisoning' for the period. Bower's impressionistic observations are given some credence by the empirical investigations of legal historians. J. S. Cockburn's study of the Kent trial records between 1560 and 1985, for example, shows that the highest rate of poisoning cases prior to the nineteenth century occurred between 1570 and 1609.[31] The *Saturday review*'s 'slumbering' eighteenth century finds support in contemporary trial records. Of over 1250 murder and attempted murder cases tried at the Central Criminal Court during the whole of the eighteenth century, only nine involved charges of poison.[32]

It is not until the middle decades of the nineteenth century – especially the 1840s and early 1850s – that the situation seems to have changed markedly. Whereas between 1829 and 1838 the Old Bailey witnessed only seven poisoning trials, in the following ten years the numbers increased more than threefold.[33] Judging by incidence, then, there is good reason to consider the middle decades of the nineteenth century as a high-point in English criminal poisoning, a conclusion reached not only by contemporaries, but by modern-day historians as well.[34] The poison 'panic' was in some sense a response to a real trend. Yet the significance attributed to the 'epidemic' of criminal poisoning in these decades cannot be explained wholly, or even primarily, by reference to numbers alone. The statistical evidence available to contemporaries, for one thing, was far from overwhelming. Official figures on homicide trials were neither collected nor published until the late 1850s, and if they had been, then they would have shown that, even at the height of the 'epidemic', poison continued to score very low by comparison with other forms of homicidal violence.[35]

However, if we shift the ground from incidence to publicly accessible representations of incidence, we can generate a more relevant set of quantitative indicators. The significant statistics from a contemporary point of view, in other words, were not actual trial rates, but how often poisoning cases were explicitly brought to public notice. To gauge this indicator, we have no better source than newspapers. Changes in patterns of reporting (in terms of frequency and content) are both indicators of, and constitutive material for, the perceptual foundation upon which the Victorian poisoning 'epidemic' was built. If we turn to *The Times* for this purpose, we notice a pattern that in some respects mirrors modern trends in trial incidence, with reports of criminal poisoning cases making an increasingly regular appearance. From only a handful between 1790 and 1810, the numbers steadily grew: fifteen between 1810 and 1819, thirty-six between 1820 and 1829, and fifty-nine between 1830 and 1839. In the 1840s, *The Times* registered a striking shift in its coverage of poisoning trials, with just over a hundred cases finding their way on to its pages. These figures become more striking still if an additional thirty-five reports from the first three years of the 1850s are factored in, yielding a total of 140 between 1840 and 1852.[36] From the perspective of an attentive *Times* reader at mid-century, then, there would be little doubt that secret poisoning was a growing problem.

But what kind of problem? How did the increasingly frequent case reports, and the comments they generated, inflect the deeper reserve of associations inherited and developed by our 'imaginative Victorian?' Reviewing the cases reported from the 1840s, four characteristics immediately stand out: three-quarters took place between individuals related by blood or marriage; of reports specifying the socio-economic standing of perpetrators and victims, a similar proportion involved members of the 'lower orders' (rural labourers, factory hands, some 'respectable' artisans and tradespeople); sixty per cent featured women as the accused parties, 37 per cent of whom were charged with poisoning their spouses; and, in nearly 70 per cent of the cases, arsenic was the chosen instrument.[37]

Poisoning as a domestic crime, of course, was not peculiar to this decade. Indeed, one of the long-standing historical resonances of poisoning is its status as a crime of intimacy. Neither is it new that poisoning was figured as a largely female crime. The characteristics historically associated with poisoners – their deceptive, cold cunning, their use of the cover of intimacy to perpetrate deadly action, for example – have, broadly speaking, been yoked under the sign of the feminine. As Margaret Hallisey has demonstrated, poisoning has in the Western literary and philosophical tradition been linked to a gendered understanding of women's attributes.[38] A wealth of examples spanning the millennia can be invoked: Eve's offer of the tainted fruit; Homer's treacherous Circe; Tacitus and Juvenal's matriarchal poisoners of Roman virtue; the venomous stepmother in Malory's Arthurian legend; and Jonson and Webster's courtly murderesses, to name only a few. This association of women with crimes of deception, and by extension to poisoning, spilled over into legal comment. The first substantive English legal treatise, the twelfth-century *Leges Henrici Primi*, treats poisoning together with witchcraft, a connection that is carried forth in subsequent centuries.[39] In the courtroom, the link was rhetorically reinforced, with the seventeenth-century jurist Lord Coke describing poisoning at a notable trial as the 'most horrible, and fearfull [*sic*] to the nature of man, and of all others [that which] can be least prevented, either by manhood or providence'.[40]

This well-entrenched association has, perhaps understandably, dominated the analyses of modern historians who have considered the topic of criminal poisoning. In such analyses there is a pronounced tendency to view poisoning as a privileged filter for capturing instances of a largely ahistorical misogynist theory in action. Yet, as important as it is to recognize the power and tenacity of the gendered imagery of poisoning, it is also vital not to neglect the historical specificity that inflects this seemingly generic set of associations. A gendered analysis of poisoning, as Sarah Currie has rightly insisted, should be able to go beyond cataloguing either cases of women poisoners or compiling examples of misogynist discourse. In other words, without neglecting the ubiquity of these gendered tropes of poisoning, it should also be understood that they will resonate differently in different historical periods, and will be used to make sense of the distinct dangers seemingly posed. In Currie's analysis, for example, the prominence of female poisoners in classical Rome can neither be explained by raw incidence (since men famously poisoned as well as females), nor by reference to a prior misogynist tradition, but by reference to a specific crisis in Roman conceptions of self-hood.[41] Hallisey's review of the poisonous women in Western literature similarly suggests historically specific features. Medieval poisoning tales, she argues, emphasized a theologically inspired condemnation of the inner corruption of woman, while downplaying the social context in which venomous women plied their trade. She notes that a shift occurred in the early modern period, in which poisonous women featured as indices of a broader social dissolution, signalled by domestic disharmony.[42]

This theme has also served as the principal lens through which historians have examined Victorian poisoning.[43] Yet this should not lead us to conclude that the gendered nature of poisoning remained a constant over this span of several centuries. If the Elizabethan Jacobean female poisoner and her Victorian cousin both represented threats to domestic harmony, they did so in ways which reflect the specific place of gender in the exercise of contemporary social and political power. From an early modern perspective, the domestic poisoner's crime was, literally, 'petty treason', following the logic of society as a vertically integrated network of sovereign males. This, Francis Dolan argues, is what drives the disproportionate interest in female domestic murderers from the mid-sixteenth to the mid-seventeenth centuries. The social and political tumult that characterized this period made commentators acutely sensitive to threats to the patriarchal order. According to Dolan, this peculiar sensitivity declined in the context of an increasingly articulated liberal critique of patriarchal order from the mid-seventeenth century onwards. With the waning of the household–kingdom homology, concern about social disorder ceased to be displaced directly on to those who threatened domestic subversion. Accordingly, accounts of 'petty treasons' like wifely poisoners (or indeed domestic servants) exercised a decreasing hold on the contemporary imagination.[44]

Victorian Britain, of course, was the exemplary site in which the liberal critique of patriarchal rule had taken root. It should come as no surprise, then, that this difference in socio-political context would result in a distinct account of the dangers represented by domestic poisoning. To be sure, the notion of a woman poisoner as a threat to patriarchy could be, and at times was, articulated by nineteenth-century commentators and participants alike. Consider, for example, Emma Hume's petition to the Queen for a reprieve of her conviction on the attempted poisoning of her husband. While denying the charge itself, Hume acknowledged, and pathetically regretted, the more general transgressions against her proper wifely role:

> when altercations have unfortunately taken place between them she has occasionally used to him disobedient, improper and threatening language of which she most sincerely repents, and which if your Majesty, in your Humanity and Kindness of Heart, should be induced to extend your royal Clemency and Mercy, she will consider it the Duty of her future Life to atone for by a dutiful and obedient conduct to her Husband.[45]

But concern with the female poisoner in 1840s was not a simple re-assertion of patriarchy in crisis. Instead, understandings of the danger were filtered through the very same liberal institutions that had displaced the patriarchal order. Like her earlier historical incarnations, as we will see below, the female poisoner of the 1840s was significant, not simply as an embodiment of a trans-historical truth, but as a point of entry into a distinctly contemporary social pathology.

Thus, while it is undoubtedly the case that poison has historically (and historiographically) been coded as feminine, the nature of this linkage and its relative importance is not fixed. Gender dysfunction was an element of, but not the exclusive referent for, Victorian reflections on the subject of criminal poisoning.[46] When a poisoning case involving a woman – especially a wife or mother – came to public attention, a ready-made narrative was immediately available to those seeking to interpret its social significance. Thus when Mary Milner was convicted of poisoning family members in 1847, *The Times* baldly described this domestic betrayal as 'a woman's crime'.[47] Yet, merely a month after declaring Milner the exemplary female assassin, *The Times* responded to John Hutchings's conviction for wife poisoning with an identical set of reflections on domestic trust betrayed: 'he had destroyed the wife of his bosom, whom

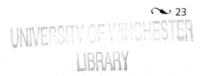

he had sworn to cherish and protect, in a most cruel manner, and while pretending to give her the cup of kindness, he had exhibited to her deliberately the cup of death'. Hutchings's conviction as a male domestic poisoner was not represented as an aberration, but instead lined up seamlessly in a list of unhappy cases which pointed to a breakdown of domestic mores. His crime was 'assassination of the worst kind – namely, that which is the result of the coldest calculation, and is committed even under the guise of affection, or by the abuse of domestic confidence'. The consequences of such crimes, irrespective of the sex of their perpetrators, were horrific to contemplate: 'Not only is life destroyed, but society is vitiated by this growing evil. The awfulness of death by guilty violence will scarcely bear a comparison with the horrible notion of the murderer at work in the family circle, pursuing his atrocious occupation through the confidence and affection with which he is regarded by his unsuspecting victim'.[48]

The interpretive framework connecting women with poison, then, formed only a part of the broader repertoire of anxieties that coalesced around the phrase 'crime of civilization'. This is not entirely surprising, given that what was generally taken as remarkable for Victorian commentators was not what linked their poisoning epidemic to the long historical record, but what made it stand out. Indeed, this is what made their insistence on passing the present incidence of poisoning through the filter of history so significant. When Victorians reached back to Roman and Stuart precedents, they were doing so in order to specify what set their own poisoning 'epidemic' apart from prior forms – situating them explicitly within the particularities of modern social institutions and relations.

These relations, moreover, were themselves subject to change. For the better part of the 1840s, the dominant image of the domestic poisoner was that of a crude and ignorant malefactor, one whose low social standing determined both motive and means. The solution to this problem followed from this typing. Poisoning was a problem that, however rich in cultural and historical connotation, could ultimately be mapped on to a grid of contemporary social analysis. It provided a unique window on to the raging 'condition of England' debate, and, in being thus located, could in turn be folded into a more generalized prescriptive vision – that of civilizing the great unwashed, bringing them under the influence of middle-class domestic virtue. By the late 1840s and early 1850s, there is a discernible shift in themes. It was here that poison came to be more commonly understood as a different sort of 'crime of civilization' – a crime signalling not civilization's partial or incomplete reach, but the limits, and paradoxes, of civilization itself. The very instruments invoked to deal with the earlier phase of crude poisoning, in other words, came to represent the ground of a new and more disturbing problem.

In the first half of the 1840s, newspapers reported on scores of domestic poisonings perpetrated in working-class households, often by wives and mothers. Through such accounts readers were able to build up a set of expectations about what they would learn in a typical poisoning case. Trial reports focused on incidental details of domestic life: the arrangements of a kitchen space, the plagues of rats and other vermin that served as the pretext for the purchase of poison. They focused on food and drink as the suspected vehicle for the poison, and thus were directed from the outside in, from the procurement of food to its preparation and ingestion. Thus, the outside world at the key moment in the trial report – when the poisonous substance passed the lips of the victim – became blocked out, the drama all unfolding within an enclosed domestic and bodily space. These narratives differed markedly from the more frequent tales of brute violence (domestic or otherwise), in which victims were instead typically expelled, bleeding and bruised, from the place of violation into an open public space.

In their emphasis on interiority, coupled with their focus on impoverished perpetrators and victims, poisoning reports provided a window on to the underside of Victorian domesticity, a way of entering the interior worlds of the social 'other'. Like reading the blue-book reports of the sanitary investigators (a related genre, to be sure), these trials participated in the construction of the underclass for a respectable readership. In these accounts, crude, promiscuous, rapacious women took centre stage: women whose husbands, children, or parents stood in the way of their selfish designs. Betty Eccles, whose dissolute ways had cost her husband his job as a respectable carter, developed an 'extraordinary and unaccountable predilection for poisoning', which, it was suspected, had claimed a previous husband and several children. Sarah Dazely, convicted of poisoning her husband and suspected of doing the same to a previous husband and child, was known in her Bedfordshire village as 'the Female Blue Beard'. Mary Gallop, who had silenced her father's opposition to an affair with a young man by means of arsenic, illustrated, in her trial judge's view, the great lengths that women might go 'to gratify their passions', while Sarah Westwood's adultery-fuelled poisoning of her husband inspired her judge to remark that he 'scarcely conceived of a crime of greater enormity or one of a deeper dye'. Sarah Freeman, suspected of sacrificing her daughter, husband, mother and brother to her 'abandoned' and 'loose' ways, provoked her local newspaper to propose a ban on the sale of poisons to women.[49]

The vulgarity displayed by these poisoners, trial reports emphasized, were matched by the crudeness with which they went about their murderous activities. Medical witnesses routinely testified to the copious amounts of arsenic they were able to recover from the bodies of victims. At the trial of Sarah Westwood, who was accused of poisoning her husband with arsenic in 1843, for example, a local surgeon remarked that 'the quantity of arsenic in the stomach was so great that it could be removed from the coats of the stomach with a spoon'.[50] Faced with such a crude and unimaginative set of poisoners, the task of the medical witness was relatively straightforward. Once suspicion had been generated and access to the body's interior secrets was secured, this brand of poisoner was readily unmasked.

Such reports, episodic and dependent on contingent events, were supplemented by more reflective, synthetic editorial comment. Editorial concern was particularly targeted at a set of suspected cases of 'systematic' poisonings carried out in rural Essex. Three cases against local women were brought to trial in 1847 and 1848, with many more reaching the stage of either police or inquest investigation. These cases seemed to indicate the existence of a sisterhood of domestic poisoners who, despite local suspicions of their murderous ways, had succeeded in dispatching scores of family members with large doses of arsenic. The first of these was Sarah Chesham, who, following highly publicized preliminary inquiries dating from the summer of 1846, was finally tried in March 1847 for poisoning two of her sons and the illegitimate son of a local farmer. Chesham was cast as a feared member of the small and isolated village of Clavering, residents 'watch[ing] her as they would a wasp, or a snake'.[51] Commenting on her case at the inquest stage, The Times highlighted two points: first, that the bodies of her victims yielded a large quantity of arsenic, sufficient to kill as many as six adults; second, that money was her motive – she had poisoned the farmer's son for a price. This poisoning for hire, moreover, was, in The Times's estimation, known to most of the inhabitants of Clavering. Chesham had lived there for years as 'a reputed poisoner – a woman whose employment was as well known as that of a nurse or a washerwoman'. Her alleged crimes bore comparison to the systematic poisoners of history – but with a crucial difference: 'Deeds which the imagination connects with the Medicis or the Gonzagas are seen at this moment naturalized in an uneducated English county'.[52]

Although Chesham's trial ended in her acquittal, the belief that systematic poisoning for profit was being pursued in a crude and barely disguised manner continued unabated. Cases which seemed to confirm the trend were reported in different parts of the country in the months following Chesham's trial, but it was when attention returned to the environs of Clavering in the following year that editorials once again took up story. In July 1848, Mary May was convicted of and executed for having administered a large dose of arsenic to her stepbrother. The following month, Hannah Southgate was charged with doing the same to her husband, allegedly with the connivance of May. Applications for permission to exhume several recently deceased husbands, moreover, were forwarded to the Home Office by officials in several neighbouring communities. These cases, collectively referred to as the 'Essex Poisoning Club', prompted agonized reflection on the cause, and the means of preventing, this 'moral epidemic far more formidable than any plague which we are likely to see imported from the East'.[53] But, in reviewing the details of the cases, it seemed as if an answer was at hand. It was true, *The Times* argued, that 'domestic tragedies are of all countries and of all times'.[54] But there existed in specific places and times social and institutional arrangements that artificially created the conditions for otherwise avoidable tragedy. Reviewing the details of the Essex cases, and those darkening Britain's criminal annals in the 1840s more generally, commentators claimed to discern a common, and avoidable, stimulus for domestic poisonings – burial clubs.

In the 1840s, burial clubs were a ubiquitous and controversial feature of life in many impoverished communities in England.[55] Growing rapidly in number during the 1830s, these were a specialized variant on friendly societies. They were small, local, informal institutions, often run from a local tavern with the publican as nominal director. For a small monthly subscription (typically between a halfpenny and a penny per week), the club undertook to pay a fixed sum intended to cover the funeral costs of members upon their death, promising an escape from the choice between the dreaded pauper's funeral and imposing a heavy financial burden on survivors. Like friendly societies, burial clubs were subjected to critical scrutiny in the early Victorian period. Run from undisciplined and potentially demoralizing spaces by men with no knowledge of actuarial science, burial clubs seemed to social and moral reformers (as well as to publicists for a rising 'modern' life insurance industry), little more than a cover for indulgence in moral and fiscal profligacy.[56]

A prominent example of this critique is Edwin Chadwick's 1843 *Report on interment in towns*, which included in its examination of 'wasteful' burial practices a denunciation of burial clubs. In one sense, Chadwick's attack formed a sub-section of his wider programme of rooting out working-class social, moral and economic indiscipline that, for him, was the cause of impoverishment. But Chadwick included in his discussion of burial-clubs a more specific charge against them – that they served as a stimulus for domestic poisonings. Two features of burial club practice made them attractive to would-be murderers, according to critics like Chadwick: first, individuals could be subscribed in as many clubs as they (or those paying the subscription) wished, thereby enabling them to receive payments beyond what was necessary to pay for the burial; and second, parents were permitted to subscribe their infant children.[57]

Drawing on a handful of recent poisoning cases in which the child victims had been members of several clubs, Chadwick insisted on the link between the ill-conceived practice of burial clubs and domestic poisoning.[58] His explanation of the phenomenon was equally in keeping with his overarching vision of a social reform based on the elimination of distortions to an otherwise functioning free-market society. The financial and institutional insecurity of burial societies, itself caused by their lack of discipline and market efficiency, led a working class intent on securing a proper burial to register family members in several clubs as a hedge against the consequences of any single club's collapse. The (initially) unintended consequence of this, Chadwick continued, was an increase in the market value of a child. 'Those aware of the moral condition of a large proportion of the population', he gloomily concluded, 'will expect that such an interest would, sooner or later, have its operation on some depraved minds to be found in every class'.[59]

For Chadwick, then, burial-club murder was an expression of the demoralizing interplay between ill-regulated institutional structures and elements of society predisposed to deviant action. What is interesting about his diagnosis, moreover, is his description of these cases as a species of perverted entrepreneurship – the natural expression of an ill-functioning market. Club murderers, according to Chadwick's logic, were not acting outside the framework of modern capitalism, but were instead making the best investment they could within the distorted market opportunities available to them.

This tension between the 'barbarism' of club poisonings and its simultaneous standing as an expression of distorted civilized sensibilities was widely echoed in contemporary commentary. Here the trope of the 'savage within', so common in this period, interacted with an identification of the 'civilized' context influencing the actions of home-grown poisoning savages. Thomas Carlyle opened his polemic against the social impact of industrialization with one of the burial-club poisoning cases highlighted in Chadwick's report. The case involved two impoverished Stockport families charged with poisoning several of their children for burial money. In its extensive coverage of the case, *The Times* declared this a 'hitherto unheard of crime', seeing it as an import from the accused's native Ireland. For Carlyle, this notion of foreignness was little more than a facile exercise in marginalization: 'In the British land', he insisted,

> a human Mother and Father, of white skin and professing the Christian religion, had done this thing; ... A human Mother and Father had said to themselves, What shall we do to escape starvation? We are deep sunk here, in our dark cellar, and help is far ... The Stockport Mother and Father think and hint: Our poor little starveling Tom, who cries all day for victuals, who will see only evil and not good in this world: if he were out of misery at once; he well dead [*sic*], and the rest of us perhaps kept alive? It is thought, hinted; at last it is done.[60]

Other critics worked the horrors of burial-club poisonings into their diagnoses of modern social ills. Benjamin Disraeli's dramatic intervention in the 'condition of England' debate, *Sybil*, drew attention to club murder as a disturbingly home-grown phenomenon: 'infanticide', he wrote, was practised 'as extensively and legally in England, as on the banks of the Ganges'.[61] The novel also highlighted the thoroughly native calculative logic at work in such cases. When an impoverished mother is faced with demands for a loan repayment, she offers half up-front, promising that the rest would follow: 'we shall have a death in our family soon: this poor babe can't struggle on much longer. It belongs to two burial clubs: that will be three pounds from each, and after the drink and the funeral, there will be enough to pay all our debts, and put us all square'.[62] Harriet Martineau, like her fellow devotee of political economy, Chadwick, identified market distortions (in this case those consequent on the poor laws) as a leading cause of 'wholesale child-murder for the sake of profits from burial clubs, and the poisonings which sweep off whole families'. This, Martineau added, was what gave modern poisoners their distinctive character: they are 'of a different order from those of whom we read in the history of past centuries', she insisted. 'They want something, – money, or a lover, or a house, or to be free of the trouble of an infant; and they put out the life which stands in the way of what they want'.[63] The noted public health reformer Joseph Kay concurred: 'a great part of the poorer classes of this country are sunk into such a frightful depth of hopelessness, misery, and utter moral degradation', he wrote in his *Social condition and education of the people in England*, 'that even mothers forget their affection for their helpless little offspring'. The result was a frighteningly perverted commodification of natural domestic sensibility, mothers killing their offspring, 'as a butcher does his lambs, in order to make money by the murder, and therewith to lessen their pauperism and misery!' Kay, typically, folds this analysis into imagery of the domestic 'other', noting with reproach that 'we are sending hundreds of thousands of our savings every year to convert and comfort the heathen, who are seldom so morally degraded'.[64] It was this same paradoxical juxtaposition of civilization and barbarity that alarmed *The Times*. Burial-club poisonings showed that 'the worst scandals of barbarism are revived and surpassed by those of civilization. To the brutality of the savage', it pointedly observed, 'is added the mercenary calculations of a civilized age'. This brute/civilized amalgam poisoned to gratify a crass and ill-governed consumerism, destroying 'on sober calculation, to buy a few days' holyday, a dress or two, and some superfluous comforts'.[65]

This recurrent theme of a calculating domestic barbarity at work from within the bosom of civilization expressed a profound anxiety. But, on the other hand, tying domestic poisoning to burial clubs also served as a form of containment. With their relentless focus on the actions of impoverished, venal, backward domesticity, middle-class reformers could simultaneously acknowledge the problem and posit a resolution fully in keeping with their own moral and economic sensibilities. To be sure, these crimes reflected badly on the materialism of the day: 'it is one of the scandals of civilization that it sacrifices nature to schemes of ambition and aggrandizement', *The Times* observed. But the scandal was contained sociologically. It was to be found amongst those 'uncared-for, unvisited, unsought, and unknown; buried in sensuality and hardened by want' – precisely those whom the full benefits of modern civilization had yet to reach. According to this analysis, then, the problem of domestic poisoning, while frightful, carried with it a prescriptive resolution: *more* civilization, spread though an intensified domestic missionary project to be undertaken by those already enjoying its fruits. *The Times* concluded its most detailed editorial on burial-club poisonings with the following ray of hope: 'Say what satirists will of the vulgarity of the middle classes, the fireside in that rank of life is the home of domestic virtues, and, as a general rule, may teach some good lessons to the ranks both above and below'.[66]

An ascendant middle-class morality, then, was the best hope of vanquishing the contemporary domestic poisoner. Crude in her method, circumscribed by her material impoverishment, she was an embarrassment in an age of refinement, to be sure, but not a contradiction of it. She could be overcome, moreover, by the better marshalling of the resources of modern civilization. This solution, it should be noted, had an administrative as well as a moral dimension. The activities of the Essex 'club poisoners' were seized upon by those calling for reform of what they considered the lax system of inquiry into suspicious or unexpected deaths operating in England and Wales. For critics like William Farr, head of the General Register Office's statistical branch, and Thomas Wakley, the reformist journalist, MP and coroner, the fact that the alleged crimes of Chesham, May, and their ilk had extended undetected over many years provided incontrovertible proof of the need for more systematic medical participation in managing deaths. Farr and Wakley repeatedly drew attention to the fact that the magistrates of the Essex county bench had hampered investigations by local coroners by refusing to pay for inquests in cases which were not, on the surface, attributable to violence or to criminal action. A more modern regime of death certification and investigation, then, would complement the project of moral reform.[67]

This moral and administrative framework of containment, however, was called into question by a concern increasingly voiced in social, legislative and scientific commentary that the dangers of poison were actually greater than crude, uncivilized venality. By the end of the decade, and well into the 1850s, a new threat was conceived of, one which had profound implications for the view of civilization and progress as a way of resolving the problem. Here the anxiety about poisoning became a self-reflexive one, the complacent containment of poison as a crime of atavistic women becoming caught up in a more entangled debate about the dangers of civilized social relations themselves. The nature of this shift, and its implications for poison as a topic of social and scientific concern, will be considered in detail in chapter 4. At this point, I merely wish to highlight one core element: a purported development in the means adopted by poisoners to dispatch their victims. Poisoners, according to leading lay and medico-legal commentators, were becoming increasingly sophisticated, eschewing single, large doses in favour of small doses over an extended period of time. This new form of poisoning, signalling a calculating patience on the part of the malefactor, and a deviousness aided in no small part by modern scientific knowledge, constituted for commentators a fresh challenge to the project of containing the criminal use of poison.

This transformation of the poisoner is best captured in the career trajectory attributed to Sarah Chesham. Chesham, as we have seen, had been at the centre of the notorious Clavering poisoning case of 1847, a case which had focused concern about the rising 'epidemic' of domestic poisoning stimulated by burial clubs. Acquitted at her first trial, Chesham returned to the criminal dock in 1851, this time charged with the murder of her husband, Richard. But there was a significant difference between the evidence adduced at the second trial, leading those framing the charge to voice private and public unease. In response to local magistrates' request for an opinion on the wisdom of proceeding to trial, for example, the Treasury Solicitor (whose duty was to advise on charges brought in the public's name) expressed reservations, observing that 'the material testimony certainly is not so decisive of the cause of Death as could be wished'. A similar opinion was offered by Alfred Swaine Taylor, the Crown's main expert witness who had also testified at Chesham's first trial: 'Morally speaking there can be little doubt of arsenic having been the cause of these intermittent attacks of illness but there is a want of that strong *medical proof* which is necessary for conviction'.[68]

The reason for these official doubts was as simple as it was disturbing. It appeared that Chesham had developed as a poisoner, and had begun to use arsenic with a deadly combination of patience and subtlety. At the trial, Taylor explained Chesham's transformation in this way: 'the arsenic must have been administered in small doses, not at all calculated to produce death at once, and when the administration of the poison was relinquished for a time the man got better'. The effect of the continual administration of small doses of arsenic, he explained, 'would be to gradually cause the powers of the body to languish, and would thus tend to develop any constitutional malady, such as consumption, that might be in the system'.[69]

Chesham's alleged adoption of a slow method of poisoning placed a number of obstacles in the way of detection. It meant, for one thing, that no large deposit of poison would be discoverable in the body after death, and further, that poisoning over an extended period of time might easily be mistaken for – or even stimulate, as Taylor's statement suggested – a natural constitutional malady. Both these points were raised in post-trial comment. Having eschewed her previous 'coarse and unscientific' methods, *The Times* observed, Chesham had stretched science's powers of detection to their very limits. As she had poisoned her husband 'at intervals and in small doses, consuming him by slow tortures', there was 'so little arsenic in his body that its presence was scarcely discoverable by the most searching tests of chymistry'.[70]

By the close of the 1840s, then, society seemed to be facing a new poisoning threat, one that placed a greater burden on the existing means of prevention. The advent of subtle poisoning, for one thing, meant that the mere reform of routine inquiries into unexplained deaths would not suffice. To counter 'scientific' poisoning, a more rigorous science of detection was required. As Taylor had noted in an 1847 *London medical gazette* editorial:

> Toxicologists are now compelled to exert their powers of discrimination upon a class of cases the true nature of which is far less readily distinguishable than was that of the instances where the obvious character of the symptoms, together with the marked traces of poisonous action discovered on post-mortem examination, usually left not the slightest doubt either of the character of the crime which had been perpetrated, or of the means by which it had been effected.[71]

Yet, Taylor and others acknowledged, toxicology had itself had a hand in creating the new threat. Previously crude poisoners like Chesham had learned their new artistic ways by studying at the feet of modern toxicology, either directly from their experience of the courtroom, or by the detailed accounts of trials found in the daily papers. Toxicology, in this sense, was part responsible for a class of poisoning autodidacts. But another, and still more terrifying, danger lurked: that of the poisoner whose science derived not from chance courtroom experience, but from purposefully, systematically, and professionally acquired knowledge. Casting a worried look over the emerging 'modern assassin', who 'adapts his expedients to the refinement of the age, bringing to his aid the appliances of science', the *Pharmaceutical journal* expressed grave doubts about toxicology's capacity to counter a truly scientific poisoner: 'To frustrate these schemes of the educated and accomplished villain would be difficult – perhaps impossible'.[72] The next two chapters will focus on the efforts made by toxicologists to rise to their possibly 'impossible' task.

Notes

1 Thomas de Quincey, 'On murder considered as one of the fine arts', *Blackwood's Edinburgh magazine*, 21 (1827), pp. 199–213, p. 209.
2 'Murder and science', *Leader* (27 August 1859), pp. 985–6; *The Times* (23 August 1860), p. 8.
3 Leslie Stephen, 'The decay of murder', *Cornhill magazine*, 20 (1869), pp. 722–33, p. 725.
4 *Ibid.*, pp. 726–7.

5 'The crime of the age', *Illustrated times* (2 February 1856), pp. 64–5, p. 64.

6 Thomas Babington Macaulay, 'Machiavelli' (orig. 1827), in *Essays, critical and miscellaneous*, 2 vols (London: J. M. Dent and Sons, 1931), 2, p. 17.

7 I am grateful to Dr Robert Di Napoli for bringing this to my attention.

8 See, e.g. Mariangela Tempera, 'The rhetoric of poison in John Webster's Italianate plays', in Michele Marrapodi, J. Oenselaars, Marcello Cappuzzo and L. Falzon Santucci (eds), *Shakespeare's Italy: functions of Italian locations in Renaissance drama* (Manchester: Manchester University Press, 1997), pp. 229–50, Julie Sanders, *Ben Jonson's theatrical republics* (Basingstoke: Macmillan, 1998), and especially Alastair Bellany, *The politics of court scandal in early modern England* (Cambridge: Cambridge University Press, 2002).

9 Edward Gibbon, *The history of the decline and fall of the Roman Empire*, 3 vols (London: A. Strahan and T. Cadell, 1789), 3, p. 67; John Millar, *The origin of the distinction of ranks* (London: John Murray, 1779), p. 103.

10 Norman Vance, *The Victorians and ancient Rome* (Oxford: Blackwell, 1997).

11 George Henry Liddell, *History of Rome* (1855), cited in 'Liddell's *History of Rome*', *Blackwood's Edinburgh magazine* 79 (1856), pp. 249–65, p. 261.

12 Vance, *The Victorians*, especially pt I.

13 Thomas Babington Macaulay, 'John Hampden', *Essays* 1, p. 110. Sporus and Locusta were notorious figures in Nero's legendarily poisonous imperial court.

14 It should be noted that this was a discourse that ran deep in the Victorian textual imagination. The imperial poisoners, Locusta, Claudius, and Agrippina, mediated by the commentaries of Juvenal, Livy, and Tacitus, and their renaissance counterparts like the Borgias and the Gonzagas, were called upon to bear historical witness to their crimes, not merely by classically minded historians, but by more obviously popular texts of the day. Newspapers from *The Times* to the *News of the world* were able to invoke them, without explanatory comment, when reporting a seemingly mundane contemporary poisoning case, as were criminal broadsheets written to commemorate (and commodify) celebrated cases. Popular novelists could similarly draw upon this well of historical association to add depth to their tales of criminality.

15 John Stuart Mill, 'Civilization', (1836) in J. M. Robson (ed.) *Collected works* 18 (London and Toronto: Routledge & Kegan Paul/University of Toronto Press, 1977), pp. 119–47, p. 131.

16 Thomas Carlyle, *Past and present* (New York: New York University Press, 1965, orig. 1843), p. 148; Matthew Arnold, *Essays*, cited in Walter Houghton, *The Victorian frame of mind* (New Haven and London: Yale University Press, 1957), p. 46.

17 *Ibid.*, p. 132. There is a large literature on the theme of anomie and modern (especially urban) civilization, including Richard Sennett, *The fall of public man* (New York: Knopf, 1977); Alexander Welch, *George Eliot and blackmail* (Cambridge, MA: Harvard University Press, 1985), especially chs 10–11;

and, for a discussion of this theme in relation to Reynolds among other mid-century authors, see Richard Maxwell, *The mysteries of Paris and London* (Charlottesville and London: University of Virginia Press, 1992).

18 G. W. M. Reynolds, *The mysteries of London*, 6 vols (London: John Dicks, 1845–48), 1, p. 148.

19 *Illustrated times*, 'The crime of the age', p. 64.

20 *The Times* (23 August 1860), p. 8.

21 *Ibid.* (3 December 1846), p. 5; (22 July 1847), p. 7; (8 September 1847), p. 6.

22 *News of the World* (30 March 1845), pp. 3–4.

23 *The Times* (31 March 1845), p. 4.

24 'Inquest on which the absurd dictum of Lord Ellenborough was pronounced', *Lancet* 1 (1842–43), pp. 362–4, p. 364; William Baker, letter to the Registrar General (1840) reprinted in Baker, *A practical compendium of the recent statutes, cases, and decisions affecting the office of coroner* (London: Butterworths, 1851), p. 382; 'Household crime', *Household words* 4 (1852), pp. 277–81, p. 277.

25 *The Times* (23 August 1860), p. 8.

26 Edward Bulwer Lytton, *Lucretia, or children of the night* (London: Routledge/Thoemmes Press, 1998, orig. 1846), p. ix.

27 Lytton, *A word to the public. By the author of 'Lucretia', etc.* (London: Saudners and Otley, 1847), pp. 46–7.

28 Lytton, *Lucretia*, pp. 49, 235.

29 'Poisoning in England', *Saturday review* 1 (1855), pp. 134–5, p. 135.

30 Barbara Hanawalt, *Crime and conflict in English communities, 1300–1348* (London and Cambridge, MA: Harvard University Press, 1979), p. 117; Richard Ireland, 'Chaucer's toxicology', *Chaucer Review* 29 (1994–95), pp. 74–91, pp. 75–7.

31 F. T. Bower, 'The audience and the poisoner of Elizabethan tragedy', *Journal of English and German philology* 36 (1937), pp. 491–504, pp. 498–9; J. S. Cockburn, 'Patterns of violence in English society: homicide in Kent, 1560–1985', *Past and present* 130 (1991), pp. 70–106, pp. 79–80. Poison cases constituted between 4 and 5 per cent of total homicides investigated during this period, as compared with an average of just under 2 per cent for the period 1560–1800. The small numbers involved (no more than three per year) makes the increase of little real significance, but of course the *Saturday review*'s 'two hundred year slumber' had little to do with its trawls through assize records.

32 Figures for the eighteenth century are based on a search of the Old Bailey proceedings online (www.oldbaileyonline.org; last accessed 16 June 2005). J. M. Beattie's research into the Surrey assizes between 1660 and 1800 confirms the comparative rarity of poisoning cases for this period. J. M. Beattie, *Crime and the courts in England, 1660–1800* (Princeton: Princeton University Press, 1986), p. 101.

33 According to Thomas Rogers Forbes, twenty-three cases were tried at the Old Bailey between 1839 and 1848, seventeen between 1849 and 1858, and seven between 1859 and 1868. Forbes, *Surgeons at the Bailey: English forensic medicine to 1878* (London and New Haven: Yale University Press, 1985), p. 128. In England and Wales overall, according to a parliamentary return, around 170 persons in England and Wales were tried for poisoning or attempted poisoning between 1839 and 1849, inclusive (*British parliamentary papers* 1850 [599], xlv, 447, 'Return of the number of persons, male and female, tried in the United Kingdom for murder and attempts to murder; by the administration of poison').

34 See, e.g., P. W. J. Bartrip, 'A "pennurth of arsenic for rat poison": the Arsenic Act, 1851 and the prevention of secret poisoning', *Medical history* 36 (1992), pp. 53–69.

35 Bartrip, 'A "pennurth"', p. 57, and Anne Crowther and Brenda White, *On soul and conscience: the medical expert and crime* (Aberdeen: Aberdeen University Press, 1988), p. 19, also argue that statistics cannot in themselves account for the intensity of concern about criminal poisoning at mid-century.

36 *The Times* carried reports of three-quarters of the poisoning trials listed in the parliamentary returns for the period 1839–49. Thus, while not fully comprehensive, this sample provides a solid basis upon which to examine the themes developed in journalistic accounts, and, of course, does indicate what the newspaper's audience would have been encountered as a journalistic representation of criminal poisoning trials. I am grateful to Professor Martin Wiener for alerting me to several *Times* poisoning reports that I had overlooked.

37 *The Times* reported the cases of twenty-six women who were tried for poisoning or attempting to poison their husbands during the 1840s, compared with twelve husbands. This preponderance of female spousal poisoning marked a departure from previous decades, where husbands and wives were equally represented (sixteen wives and fifteen husbands between 1820 and 1839).

38 Margaret Hallisey, *Venomous woman: fear of the female in literature* (New York, Westport and London: Greenwood Press, 1987).

39 Ireland, 'Chaucer's toxicology', p. 77. The etymological interchangeability of poison and witchcraft (*veneficium*) was a stock observation in explaining this connection. Indeed, the commonplace image of the female poisoner was invoked by those seeking to naturalize witchcraft: 'As women in all ages have been counted most apt to conceive witchcraft', the sixteenth-century investigator Reginald Scot observed, 'so also it appeareth, that they have been the first inventers, and the greatest practitioners of poisoning, and more naturallie addicted and given thereunto than men'. Reginald Scot, *The discoverie of witchcraft* (London and Arundel: Centaur Press, 1964, orig. 1584), pp. 112–13.

40 Sir Edward Coke, *The third part of the institutes of the laws of England: concerning high treason, and other pleas of the crown, and criminal causes*, cap. 7, 48 (London: W. Clarke: 1809).

41 Sarah Currie, 'Poisonous women and the unnatural history of Roman culture', in Maria Wyke (ed.), *Parchments of gender* (Oxford: Oxford University Press, 1998), pp. 147–67; Hallisey, *Venomous woman*, ch. 2.

42 *Ibid.*, pp. 19–20.

43 See, e.g., George Robb, 'Circe in crinoline: domestic poisonings in Victorian England', *Journal of family history*, 22:2 (1997), pp. 176–90, and Judith Knelman, *Twisting in the wind: the murderess and the English press* (Toronto, Buffalo and London: University of Toronto Press, 1998).

44 Several other historians have noted the over-representation of women as murderers in general in early modern popular texts, e.g. Francis Dolan, *Dangerous familiars: representations of domestic crime in England, 1550–1700* (Ithaca and London: Cornell University Press, 1994), espescially ch 1, Peter Lake, 'Deeds against nature: cheap print, Protestantism and murder in early seventeenth-century England', in Kevin Sharpe and Peter Lake (eds), *Culture and politics in early Stuart England* (Basingstoke: Macmillan, 1993, pp. 257–83), and Martin Wiener, 'Alice Arden to Bill Sikes: changing nightmares of intimate violence in England, 1558–1869', *Journal of British studies* 40 (2001), pp. 184–212. Vanessa McMahon's recent study of early modern homicide indicates that female poisoners follow this pattern: she finds more male than female poisoners (in both relative and absolute terms) in the legal files she has consulted, but far more female than male poisoners in contemporary chapbooks and broadsheets. McMahon, *Murder in Shakespeare's England* (London: Hambledon and London, 2004). I am grateful to Dr McMahon for allowing me to see portions of her manuscript prior to publication.

45 The National Archives (TNA): Public Record Office, London (hereafter PRO) HO 18/204/25: Emma Hume petition (6 August 1844).

46 Consider, for instance, the record of trial accounts. Although a stock historical figure, the female poisoner only began to dominate *Times* trial reports in the 1840s. Between 1820 and 1839, 56 per cent of its poisoning trial reports featured men, while the gender ratio amongst spousal poisonings was virtually 1:1. During the 1840s, by contrast, 60 per cent of *The Times* reports involved women accused, while, in 68 per cent of its spousal poisoning trials, wives stood as the accused. In her survey of 540 poisoning cases between 1750 and 1914, Katherine Watson finds a near gender parity amongst the accused, with only 51 per cent involving women. This figure shifts when she restricts her sample to charges involving murder, attempted murder, and manslaughter (56 per cent female). Amongst the 134 spousal poisoners in her survey, 56 per cent were wives. Katherine Watson *Poisoned lives: English poisoners and their victims* (London and New York: London and Hambeldon, 2004), pp. 45, 47. As George Robb has pointed out, in evaluating all such figures it should

be remembered that since males were the accused in the overwhelming number of total homicide trials, women were disproportionately represented in the ranks of homicidal poisoners. Robb also states that while 90 per cent of Victorian spousal killers were men, only 5 per cent of murderous husbands used poison, as compared with 55 per cent of murderous wives. Robb, 'Circe', p. 177.

47 *The Times* (9 August 1847), p. 6.
48 *Ibid.* (24 September 1847), p. 7.
49 *Ibid.* (4 October 1842), p. 4; (8 August 1843), p. 7; (10 December 1844), p. 7; (30 December 1844), p. 7; (30 December 1843), p. 7; (13 January 1845), p. 3.
50 *Ibid.* (30 December 1843), p. 7.
51 *Ibid.* (21 September 1846), p. 4.
52 *Ibid.*
53 *Ibid.* (22 September 1848), p. 4.
54 *Ibid.* (20 September 1848), p. 4
55 For more on burial clubs, see P. H. J. H. Gosden, *Self-help: voluntary associations in the nineteenth century* (London: Batsford, 1973), ch. 5, and Eric Hopkins, *Working-class self-help in nineteenth-century England* (London: University College London Press, 1995), pt 1; for the link between burial clubs and infanticide, see George Behlmer, *Child abuse and moral reform in England, 1870–1908* (Palo Alto, CA: Stanford University Press, 1982), and Lionel Rose, *The massacre of innocents: infanticide in Britain 1800–1939* (London: Routledge & Kegan Paul, 1986). I thank Professor Behlmer for sharing his thoughts with me on this topic.
56 For an illuminating discussion of this trend in the case of friendly societies, see Elizabeth Wallace, 'The needs of strangers: friendly societies and insurance societies in late eighteenth-century England', *Eighteenth-century life* 24 (2000), pp. 53–72.
57 As Behlmer and Rose note, there were rules against these practices, but the informal and unregulated nature of burial clubs meant that they not strictly enforced.
58 Chadwick himself cited four cases since 1839. By the end of the 1840s the list of core exemplary cases cited by commentators had grown to about ten. Edwin Chadwick, 'Supplementary report on the result of a special inquiry into the practice of interment in towns', *British parliamentary papers*, 1843 [509.], xii. 395, 64–9; *The Times* (18 January 1849), p. 3.
59 Chadwick, 'Supplementary report', 64.
60 Carlyle, *Past and present*, pp. 9–10.
61 Benjamin Disraeli, *Sybil, or the two nations* (London: Longmans, Green and Co., 1871, orig. 1845), bk 2, ch. 10, p. 113
62 *Ibid.*, bk 3, ch. 3, p. 182.
63 Harriet Martineau, *The history of England during the thirty years' peace, 1816–46*, 3 vols (London: Charles Knight, 1849), 1, pp. 560, 559. Martineau

also connected poisoning to burial club abuse in 'A death watch worth dreading', *Once a week* 2 (1859–60), pp. 18–22.

64 Joseph Kay, *The social condition and education of the people in England*, 2 vols (London: Longman, Brown, Green and Longmans, 1850), 1, p. 447.

65 *The Times* (12 December 1853), p. 6.

66 *Ibid.*

67 Note that the difficulties in dealing with this class of poisoner, for the likes of Farr and Wakley, lay not in the complexities of toxicology – since, once the cases were brought under investigation, the large amounts of arsenic were easy to find – but with a lax system of preliminary inquiry which failed to identify cases requiring investigation. For more on this, see Ian Burney, *Bodies of evidence: medicine and the politics of the English inquest, 1830–1926* (Baltimore and London: Johns Hopkins University Press, 2000), especially ch. 2.

68 PRO TS 23/513: Case respecting the suspected poisoning of Richard Chesham by Sarah his wife. Emphasis original.

69 *The Times* (7 March 1851), p. 6.

70 *Ibid.* (8 March 1851), p. 4.

71 'On the increase of the crime of secret poisoning', *London medical gazette* 4 (n.s.) (1847), pp. 191–4, p. 192. Taylor was editor of the *LMG* from 1844 to 1851.

72 'Secret poisoning', *Pharmaceutical journal* 9, 1849–50, p. 201.

2

Disciplining poison

Among the myriad of instruments available for perpetrating criminal violence against the nineteenth-century body, poison was the only one thought to require its own dedicated expert. Against the scourge of criminal poisoning, it was the toxicologist who stood out as its most conspicuous counterweight. The richness of poison's cultural terrain, its deep historical and imaginative resonances, presented the science of poison detection with both opportunities and obstacles. On the one hand, it provided would-be experts with a highly visible platform upon which to demonstrate their wares. Yet its singular notoriety as an instrument of criminal violence meant that poison did not present itself to its presumed experts as an exclusively scientific object. For this reason, the attempt to discipline poison, to translate the rich public discourse explored in the previous chapter into a scientific one, was an essential feature in efforts to construct a 'modern' toxicology.

This task had several distinct components that can be analyzed usefully in terms of 'containment' – containment of poison conceptually, operationally and legislatively. Conceptual containment involved re-writing the boundaries between poison's exotic past and its properly scientific present. Operationally, it entailed formulating an identity for poison that would position it as a suitable object of expert intervention. Legislatively, it required a further definitional identity, one that made poison amenable to a regime of regulation and prohibition.

Before considering these overlapping projects, however, we ought to briefly survey the prevailing state of British legal medicine generally, and of toxicology in particular. Medical jurisprudence in Britain, in the view of both contemporaries and historians, was a singularly undisciplined subject in the early decades of the nineteenth century, with commentators lamenting its comparatively weak position as a recognized field of knowledge and practice. It was not until the second decade of the nineteenth century that a systematic British work on the subject was published – earlier works being little more than selective glosses on a continental treatise tradition already well established by the sixteenth century.[1] The subject fared no better institutionally. While university positions had been established throughout continental Europe in the previous century, the first British chair of medical jurisprudence was not established until 1807, when the University of Edinburgh appointed the physician Andrew Duncan Jr as its first professor. Duncan's appointment, as Anne Crowther and Brenda White have shown, was of limited impact. As a subject, medical jurisprudence had a marginal place within the university curriculum, not being a compulsory part of any degree course offered. Duncan's approach to the subject, moreover, emphasized a cameralist 'State Medicine', and in his twelve-year tenure he did little to develop a systematic study of medical jurisprudence as applied to the civil and criminal courtroom.[2]

In 1822, the professorship's place as a minor instrument of patronage seemed set to continue with the appointment of Robert Christison, the twenty-five-year-old son of a much-respected and recently retired Edinburgh professor of Latin. Yet, within a decade, Christison, an Edinburgh medical-school graduate with a special interest in chemistry, had emerged as Britain's first recognized authority on medical jurisprudence. Intent on developing its standing as a body of knowledge applied in the legal courtroom, Christison sought to ground the subject institutionally as well as conceptually. His course was incorporated into the medical curriculum, first as an optional subject in 1825, and in 1833 as a requirement for all graduates. This, along with Edinburgh's Royal College of Surgeons' decision to require attendance at a course of medical jurisprudence for all those intending to sit its qualifying examination, boosted class numbers, which increased ninefold during Christison's decade in the post. Christison also succeeded in positioning himself as a practitioner and theorist of national and even international standing, using his editorial position on the influential *Edinburgh medical and surgical journal* as a platform for commenting on developments in the field.[3] When, following his involvement in the sensational Burke and Hare trial, Christison was appointed medico-legal adviser to the Crown in Scotland in 1829, his place as the leading British exponent of his field was secured.

In London, the other major British centre of medical education, the process of institutionalization was slower.[4] Although lectures on medical jurisprudence were given on a sporadic basis from the early 1820s, it was not until 1828 that the fledgling University of London established

England's first chair in the subject, appointing the Edinburgh graduate, John Gordon Smith. Smith's professorship was far from secure, however. His salary was almost entirely dependent on student fees, yet his capacity to attract students was hampered by the fact that neither of the main medical licensing bodies (the Society of Apothecaries and the Royal College of Surgeons) required instruction in medical jurisprudence for their diplomas. Smith thus spent much of his three-year tenure petitioning various bodies, including his own university court of examiners, the Society of Apothecaries, and the Home Office, in an effort to gain recognition for the subject.

Smith was joined in this effort by other would-be lecturers in the field, and by elements of the reformist medical press, lead by Thomas Wakley's *Lancet*. Wakley embraced the cause of medical jurisprudence as part of a broader campaign to displace a medicine 'corrupted' institutionally and conceptually through patronage and tradition. Medical jurisprudence, in principle, provided an exemplary demonstration of the importance of a progressive approach to medical education and accreditation: as a synthetic body of knowledge embracing physiology, pathology, and chemistry, it required a solid grounding in what were being described as the basic medical sciences; and as a high-profile exercise in social intervention, it demonstrated the potential for properly trained practitioners to contribute accredited expertise to the wider aims of good governance.[5] Once freed from its present, shambolic form, in which intellectually and institutionally unsupported medical witnesses were routinely humiliated in the adversarial context of the courtroom, medical jurisprudence might come to symbolize the legitimate deployment of a universalist, meritocratic, and socially engaged scientific expertise.

This campaign achieved a measure of success when the Society of Apothecaries agreed that, as of January 1831, all candidates for its increasingly popular licence (LSA) had to provide certificates of attendance at a three-month course of medical jurisprudence.[6] Although criticized by reformers (firstly, because certificates were only accepted from medical schools recognized by the 'corrupt' Royal College of Physicians, and secondly because the subject was not itself an examinable element of the LSA),[7] the Society's policy did have the immediate effect of increasing the number of lectureships in medical jurisprudence attached to metropolitan institutions of medical education. Within a few years, most of these were offering a course in the subject, taught generally by young graduates of their own institutions seeking a foothold on the institutional ladder. While several of these metropolitan lecturers would later establish reputations for themselves in other fields, only one of this first cohort made a significant impact on the field of medical jurisprudence itself.[8] This was Alfred Swaine Taylor, about whom much will be said in the coming pages.[9] A student of Guy's Medical School, Taylor had only recently attained membership of the Royal College of Surgeons, when in 1831, at the age of twenty-five, he was named as Guy's lecturer in medical jurisprudence. Taylor's position, like that of his fellow medical jurists, although sometimes referred to as a 'professorship,' was a marginal one within the school, commanding neither a guaranteed salary, tenure of appointment, nor dedicated facilities for pursuing his subject.[10]

Both Christison in Edinburgh and Taylor in London, then, commenced their work in medical jurisprudence on shaky institutional foundations. For the viability of the subject as well as their own financial well-being, they needed to generate interest amongst students, medical professionals, legal and governmental officials, and the public. It is significant that in this context both chose to focus on toxicology as their field of special interest. Several reasons might be given to explain this emphasis. In their medical studies they had pursued interests in chemistry, a subject which itself attracted a great deal of interest among students and the public more generally in the early decades of the nineteenth century.[11] For Christison, the combination of novelty and inherent public fascination made the medico-legal study of poison seem a promising means to achieve his promotional ends. It was, he recalled in an 1851 address, a field 'almost untrodden by British cultivators, yet at the same time more full perhaps of varied interest than any other, better fitted at all events to attract general notice'.[12] Christison's recollections on the novelty of his toxicological interests were perhaps overstated, as the (admittedly limited) existing British medico-legal literature typically devoted more pages to poison than to any other single topic. Yet with the publication of Christison's *Treatise on poisons* in 1829 – the first British text devoted exclusively to the subject – toxicology was undoubtedly set on a new footing as the most well-defined and recognizable representative of British medical jurisprudential knowledge.[13]

Knowledge, in Christison's case, is the keyword here, his approach to the subject placing strong emphasis on its status as a developing experimental field. In addition to reporting on the results of his own toxicological research, Christison's text provided readers with copious references to the latest developments from the leading European laboratories, and he took careful note of work on poison with applications beyond the courtroom. Indeed, he devoted the first chapter of his treatise entirely to a review of physiological and pharmacological work undertaken by continental experimentalists like Magendie, Pelletier and Caventou, and – closer to home – by Brodie, and Morgan and Addison.

By contrast, Taylor's *On Poisons in relation to medical jurisprudence* (1848) was of a more limited scope, setting itself the task of providing the information requisite for medical men who, in the course of their professional work, might be called upon to testify in a case of suspected poisoning. This text was structured less by reference to laboratory results than by legal precedents taken from recent court cases. Thus, for example, Taylor reined in discussion of contemporary experiments into the action of poison, and their significance for understanding both basic animal physiology and chemical therapeutics, describing them as 'highly interesting in a physiological and pathological view; but . . . not of much importance to a medical jurist'.[14]

What *was* of importance to the medical jurist, Taylor asserted, was a body of practical knowledge for use in cases coming under legal scrutiny. An important reason for this emphasis stems from the system under which English medico-legal cases were investigated. In contrast to Scotland and to most continental countries, England had a highly decentralized system for inquiring into suspicious death. Initial inquiries came under the jurisdiction of the local coroner, who was empowered to commission a post-mortem investigation, with or without chemical analysis. In the vast majority of cases involving such medico-legal examination, it was a local medical man – often the deceased's own attendant – who carried them out.[15] Given this investigative structure (which was itself the subject of much criticism by medico-legal modernizers), Taylor's principal constituency was the ordinary practitioner who, at any time, might be called upon to represent toxicological science in the courtroom. The dissemination of this information, Taylor asserted in the preface to *On poisons*, was of particular importance in the context of an England that at mid-century required a bulwark against what he insisted was a real social menace: 'The crime of poisoning has been of late so fearlessly on the increase', he observed, 'that it seems essential for the proper administration of justice, and for the security of society, to collect and arrange in a convenient form for reference, those important medical facts in relation to death from poison'.[16]

Toxicology, then, had at least two professional constituencies: first, ordinary practitioners, mainly local surgeons and apothecaries, who conducted post-mortems and chemical analyses in the bulk of suspected poisoning cases; and second, experts like Christison and Taylor, who represented toxicology in cases of 'special difficulty'.[17] It is worth noting here the implications of this fact for what will be referred to as 'toxicological expertise' in the coming pages. Poison cases did not take evidence of specialist chemical analysts as a matter of course. Indeed, of the cases reported by *The Times* from the 1840s and 1850s, fewer than one in ten trials involved expertise beyond a local medical practitioner. Yet, in virtually every instance, these cases did feature some display of toxicological knowledge. Where no chemist or toxicologist had been called in, ordinary practitioners delivered the results of analyses that they themselves had performed. In doing so, they had recourse to a collective body of knowledge, filtered down to them through authorities like Christison and Taylor, and which they often explicitly invoked. In this sense, toxicology was present at all poison trials, and, by extension, figured as a form of expertise possessed, if not always represented, by a community of dedicated practitioners: a community recognized both by medico-legal commentators and the public who looked to them for protection against the secret poisoner. It is this toxicology – invoked in the intertwined public and professional discourses on criminal poisoning and its prevention – that features most prominently in the coming pages.

With this background in mind, we can now return to the theme of 'containment' suggested at the start of the chapter. For those seeking to set toxicology on a modern footing, institutional reform had to be complemented by a more diffuse set of transformations through which poison might be positioned as, first and foremost, an object of scientific intervention. Let us begin with the daunting task of taming poison's unruly past. This was a task, to be sure, that confronted all those who in the early nineteenth century strove towards disciplinary specialism. But, for would-be poison specialists, the past was a particularly important object of intervention because, as we have seen, it was such a core feature of Victorian discussions on poisoning. To make toxicology a properly scientific field of study, this multi-layered public discourse had to be subsumed under the rubric of sober fact.

This is a process that can be discerned at a variety of levels, beginning with the shifting origins attributed to the word 'toxicology' itself. Although used in continental texts from the last quarter of the eighteenth century, the *OED* gives as its first English-language example of the term an entry in Robert Hooper's 1799 *Medical dictionary*, defining toxicology as 'a dissertation on poisons'. The derivation of the term, in Hooper's account, was from the Greek roots 'discourse' and 'arrow or bow', the latter, Hooper explained, 'because the darts of the antients [*sic*] were usually besmeared with some poisonous substance'.[18] Twenty years later, however, the same *Dictionary* defined toxicology as 'the study of poisons', and provided it with a revised etymological pedigree that replaced ancient arrows with the more straightforward root 'a poison'.[19] The entry for toxicology in Forbes's 1836 *Cyclopaedia*, which offered the same definition and etymology as the later edition of Hooper, provided a rationale for this decision: the Greek root for 'poison' was commonly attributed to the word for 'bow', it explained,

> either, as Dioscorides says, because barbarians were accustomed to anoint their arrows with poison; or, as others think, because poison destroys life as rapidly and certainly as an arrow from the bow; or, lastly, because Hercules dipped his arrows in the (poisonous) blood of the hydra. Some, however, are of opinion – and I own this to me seems the most probable conjecture – that the word . . . is the name of a poisonous plant, growing in Syria or Africa.[20]

The attributes of plants, rather than ancient myth, for the up-to-date etymologist, seemed a more likely foundation for deriving 'the study of poisons'. The modern toxicologist would, of course, have fully concurred.

Numerous other examples could be cited in which contemporary writers sought to disengage poison from an unusable, mythic past.[21] But for our purposes, one theme stands out above all others – legendary tales of 'slow poison'. In the accounts of the celebrated poisoners of the classical and Renaissance periods that underpinned the Victorian image of poison's past, their mastery of this subtle art was a staple feature. Slow poison, in this tradition, had a precise meaning, referring to substances that acted not merely by incremental and undetectable degree, but more importantly by a degree predetermined by the skill of the poisoner. A proper slow poison, in short, was one that, once introduced into the body, could kill at a future time specified by its author.

The question as to the factual existence of 'slow poisons' had been a perennial theme in poison literature. In ancient and medieval accounts, this was an issue that linked the art of poisoning with the occult. As Lyn Thorndike observes, poisoning since ancient times has been linked with sorcery and magic. In Greek and Latin 'poison' and 'sorcery', as well as 'drug' and 'magical potion', were denoted by the same word, and mysterious deaths might equally be attributed to one or the other.[22] Poison's mode of action was similarly suspended between natural and occult principles. Amongst the ancient Greeks and Romans, Clyde Pharr explains, persons could be bewitched or killed by *pharmakon* or *venenum*, which could be deployed at a distance, and operated not merely through its own internal properties but in association with secret incantations, charms, and magical ceremonies.[23] This conceptual doubling, furthermore, found its expression in ancient legal theory and practice. Plato's *Laws* distinguished between two forms of poison, one working 'according to natural law', the other working by 'sorceries and incantations', while the *Institutes* of Justinian grouped sorcerer–poisoners under the same cognate category.[24] This association, as Richard Ireland demonstrates, was echoed in English law, the twelfth-century *Leges Henrici Primi* treating poison together with witchcraft and necromancy, a connection reinforced by subsequent statutes.[25]

Slow poison was a matter of live authoritative dispute in the early modern period, in England as well as on the continent. Thomas Spratt relates investigations undertaken at the Royal Society on the alleged subtle properties of New World poisons, with members debating whether New World natives could make preparations that could 'lie several days, months, years, according as they will have it, in a man's body, without doing him any hurt, and at the end kill him without missing half an hour's time'.[26] The physician William Ramesey's 1665 treatise, after reviewing the learned debate from both sides, decided against the existence of poisons 'as will kill at such a certain and prefixed time', not on the grounds of physical impossibility, but because of the imperfect state of human knowledge. 'It is not probable any man, in this life, should attain to that perfection of Knowledge', Ramesey declared, 'as to know exactly any ones [*sic*] temperature so as to prepare his medicine accordingly'.[27]

Eighteenth-century treatises devoted to the subject of poison, although retaining an interest in the topics favoured by earlier authors, demonstrated an increasing interest in naturalizing the subject. This more experimentally minded and secular account of poisoning, of course, was part of the larger effort to map phenomena previously associated with hidden, inner principles on to a more empirical grid emphasizing natural forces. The most significant English exemplar was Richard Mead's 1702 *Mechanical account of poisons*, which set out to shift the understanding of the action of poisons, from 'some Occult or Unknown Principle' to 'the known Laws of Motion'. Poisons acted by dint of physical – albeit minute – action, Mead concluded, as they contained physical particles that should be considered 'as so many sharp Knives or Daggers, Wounding and Stabbing the tender Coats of the Stomach, and thus causing excessive Pains'.[28]

Although, by the end of the eighteenth century, Mead's strictly mechanical account of the action of poisons had been replaced by a more complex physiological debate about whether poison acted via absorption (blood) or sympathy (nerves), his resolutely naturalistic explanatory frame of reference was the undisputed foundation upon which a modern toxicology was expected to build. Yet, taking the place of slow poison in English medico-legal texts as an indicator, we can see that the road to a 'disciplined' understanding of poison was not a smooth one. The Birmingham physician, George Edward Male, in the first edition of his *Epitome of juridical or forensic medicine* (the first substantive English treatise dedicated to medico-legal theory and practice) included without critical comment an account of the history of slow, subtle poisonings, noting that 'many have fallen sacrifice to this insidious treachery, when least expecting it'.[29] His second edition (1818) extends the discussion by detailing cases of slow poisoning recorded by such familiar sources as Tacitus, Theophrastus, and Quintilian. Only after this lengthy treatment does he conclude with a profession of provisional scepticism: 'Notwithstanding the above cited authorities, the existence of this class of poisons has been doubted, and the peculiar powers which they have been supposed to possess of producing their lethal effects at a remote given period, previously calculated upon, have *probably* been exaggerated by vulgar credulity'.[30]

The next significant English treatise, the physician John Ayrton Paris and the barrister Anthony Fonblanque's 1824 *Medical jurisprudence*, devoted one of its three volumes almost entirely to the subject of poison. It opened with an extended discussion of poison's 'literary history', covering canonical topics in '*occult* and *slow* poisoning' – knives poisoned on one side only, poisoned boots prepared by Oriental poison virtuosi, and the lethal properties of bullock's blood, among many others. These accounts suggested ancient knowledge of certain subtle poisons 'so extreme as to defeat the most skilful caution, and at the same time so manageable as to be capable of the most accurate graduation', enabling the malefactor to 'measure his allotted moments with the nicest precision, and to occasion his death at any period that might best answer the objects of the assassination'. Despite having run through these topics at considerable length, Paris and Fonblanque conclude by echoing Male's caution in a more declarative mode: 'such is the ambiguity of ancient writers upon this subject, and so intimately blended are all their receipts with the practices of superstition, that every research, however learned, into the exact nature of the poisons which they employed, is necessarily vague and unsatisfactory'. Slow poisoning, though perhaps once a topic for proper discussion, was lost to, and thus irrelevant for, the modern student.[31]

Early nineteenth-century medico-legal writers thus indulged in extended discussions of slow poison legend, if only to underscore its irretrievability. For Robert Christison, such efforts were distractions, and in his 1829 *Treatise on poisons* he made a more explicit attempt to preserve toxicology from the contamination of myth. Describing legitimate interest in the subject as 'purely medico-legal', Christison criticized what he saw as the continued influence of slow poison histories, not merely in the popular imagination, but in ostensibly modern medico-legal texts. He attributed this influence to a misplaced deference to their 'classic origin', or their ability to 'feed our appetite for the mysterious', and called upon a critical sensibility more appropriate to the age to disown this fanciful past: 'No one', he ventured, 'now seriously believes that Henry the Sixth was killed by a pair of poisoned gloves, or Pope Clement the Seventh by a poisoned torch carried before him in a procession, or Hercules by a poisoned robe, or that the operation of poisons can be so predetermined as to commence or prove fatal on a fixed day, and after the lapse of a definite and remote interval'. 'It is plain to every modern toxicologist', Christison concluded, that ancient poisoning artists 'owed their success rather to the ignorance of the age, than to their own dexterity'.[32]

With the publication of Alfred Swaine Taylor's *On poisons* some two decades later, the process of marginalizing slow poison seemed to have reached completion. Taylor studiously avoids any mention of celebrated historical tales, and the brief references he does make to the topic refrain from engaging in even dismissive elaboration. In keeping with his expressed aim of writing a handbook of toxicological practice, Taylor replaces indulgence in historical accounts with a relentlessly practical framework. In his hands, classical stories of historical crimes yield to sober and detailed accounts of contemporary poisoning cases drawn from the annals of the English courtroom, a place which, in his view, had no need for poison's fanciful past.

This incremental marginalization of substantive consideration of the ancient art of slow poisoning serves as a telling example of how medico-legal authors sought to disengage poison from the literary and historical imagination, and to naturalize it as the object of a modern, practical science. A related – and arguably more crucial – task involved reconstructing knowledge about the phenomenology of poisoning. In cases of suspected criminal poisoning, the most basic of all questions to be answered was whether or not the purported victim in fact died from the effects of poison. Like any claim to expert competence, toxicology required recognition of principal, if not exclusive, competence to answer such a foundational question. The poisoned body of a functioning toxicological expertise was ideally an enigma, yielding clues to its demise only to the trained interpretive eye. It is with this imperative in mind that we can return to the suggestion made in chapter 1 that the inscrutable poisoned body – that paradigmatic victim of modern criminal violence – was in significant respects a creation of nineteenth-century toxicology.

The interpretive field surrounding a poisoned body was a complex and crowded one in the early modern period. Take, for example, the following account of the suspected poisoning of the Marquess James Hamilton, whose sudden death in 1625 prompted furious speculation that he had been poisoned by the court favourite George Villiers, Duke of Buckingham. In a trenchant denunciation of Buckingham, the royal physician George Eglisham cited the external appearance of Hamilton's corpse as a telling proof of the crime:

> No sooner was he dead, when the force of the poyson had overcome the force of his body, but it began to swell in such sort, that his Thighes were swolne six times as bigge as their naturall proportion, his Belly became as bigge as the belly of an Oxe, his Armes as the naturall quantity of his Thighes, his Neck so broad as his Shoulders, his Cheekes over the top of his Nose, that his Nose could not be seen or distinguished, the skin of his forehead two fingers high swelled, the haire of his beard eye-browes and head, so farre distant from one another, as if an hundred had been taken out betweene each one; and when one did touch the haire, it came away with the skin as easily, as if one had pulled hay out of a heap of hay. He was all over his neck, breast, shoulders, armes, and browes, I say of divers colours, full of waters of the same colour, some white, some blacke, some red, some yellow, some greene, some blew, and that as well within his body as without.
>
> Also the concavities of his Liver greene, his stomach in some places a little purpurated with a blew clammy water, adhering to the sides of it. His Mouth and Nose foaming blood mixt with froath mightily, of divers colours a yarde high. Your Petitioner being sent for to visit his body, and his servants all flocking about him, saying, See, see, perfectly weeping, said he was poysoned.[33]

This account is of interest at several levels: it depicts in stark and fulsome detail the signs of poisoning plainly visible on the outside of the body; it indicates a fluid and non-hierarchical relationship between the value of internal and external marks of poisoning; and it includes without critical comment the interpretive competence of non-medical viewers of the body.

Eglisham's contemporaries would not have been surprised by any of these features, for the value of surface signs of poisoning available to the trained eye and the casual onlooker alike was a matter widely accepted in learned texts and in everyday practice. Classical authors crediting external signs included the usual suspects: Tacitus's account of the blackened body of Germanicus, Juvenal and Livy's similarly graphic depiction of the bodies of poisoned Roman senators, for instance. Medical writers could also draw on appropriate classical authority. Culpeper and his colleagues, writing several decades after Eglisham's tract, included amongst the 'common signs' of poisoning 'a swollen tongue, black and inflamed lips, swollen belly, and body often, with spots', citing Galen's dictim that 'if his body be blew or blackish, or of divers colours, or stink, they say he is poysoned'.[34] As Malcolm Gaskell's study of early modern English trial records demonstrates, this expectation that the poisoned body would betray surface marks of unnatural violation operated in practice as well as in theory. He cites, for example, a 1610 Star Chamber case in which a Gloucestershire woman had been given a poison 'soe vennamous and stronge, as that her boddie did in such sorte swell as that it was therew[i]th lyke to burste', and a 1677 Cambridgeshire trial which heard the testimony of a woman who, on laying out the body of the supposed victim, determined that 'hee did not dye a naturall death for that [his] members were extraordinarily swel[le]d and very black'.[35]

Although, judging by trial transcripts, reliance on external signs as indicators of poisoning had begun to recede in the eighteenth century in favour of gross anatomical indicators discernible on post-mortem examination, early nineteenth-century medical witnesses continued to adduce surface appearance as part of their evaluation of a poisoning charge. In the celebrated 1809 trial of Charles Angus, one medical witness stressed the lack of surface marks as grounds for refuting the charge of poisoning, while in 1816, an apothecary at the inquest on the body of Elizabeth Ward described 'a swelling of the face, and a projection of the eyes, effects which would be the result of receiving arsenic into the stomach'.[36] As late as 1848, the possibility of tracing poison at the surface level was offered as an article of popular belief. At the trial of Ann Fisher, one witness recounted her advice to the accused to administer a reduced dose to her victim on the grounds that 'if she gave him all the poison he would swell, and then it would be found out'.[37]

Early nineteenth-century medico-legal writers were in no doubt that external signs remained an important evidentiary feature of contemporary poisoning trials. As with slow poisoning, their place in the hierarchy of proof mutated over the course of successive treatises. George Male's 1816 text gave a clearly defined space for such evidence. Frothing from the mouth soon after death, he stated, was often observed, though he added that this was not peculiar to those dying by poison. The reliability of external signs was more secure in cases involving vegetable poisons, Male asserted, as bodies poisoned by these agents 'generally swell prodigiously, soon become offensive, and covered with gangrenous spots'. Paris and Fonblanque agreed that deaths involving vegetable poisons left the medical witness with an externally legible corpse, citing in evidence Juvenal's poisonous matrons parading their husbands' blackened bodies in a funeral cortège through the streets of Rome.[38]

It was again left to Robert Christison's 1829 text to launch a more thoroughgoing assault on such 'errors' of the past. 'It was at one time thought by the profession, and is still very generally imagined by the vulgar,' he observed, 'that unusual blackness or lividity of the skin, indicates death by poison generally'. Yet these could not be considered reliable signs for a modern practitioner. Since they were not always present in poisoning cases, and, since they might feature as a by-product of any number of natural diseases, they did not justify, 'in any circumstances whatever, the slightest ground of suspicion'.[39] And it is in Taylor's 1848 treatise that we see this process of textual marginalization ostensibly completed. Here, the elaborations found in earlier works are replaced by a simple declarative statement: 'In relation to external appearances', Taylor insists, 'there are none indicative of poisoning upon which we can safely rely'.[40] The formerly crowded stage of corporeal interpreters, as a matter of toxicological principle, was cleared, with the modern poison expert left to proceed unencumbered in his task of providing an authoritative reading of the poisoned body.

Yet, despite their categorical dismissal of the value of external signs for a functioning science of poison, Christison and Taylor did not entirely eschew the body's surface. First, as we will see in the following chapter, while conclusions generated through chemical analysis were held out as the most desirable form of proof in a case of suspected poisoning, there were other sources deemed worthy of consideration. Clinical symptoms observed by an attentive medical practitioner, and post-mortem signs uncovered from the body's interior at the autopsy table, most importantly, could both serve either as confirmation of chemical analysis or, where for specific reasons such analysis failed, as an alternative form of proof. In addition to these sanctioned adjuncts of toxicological analysis, Christison advised his readers to attend to popular conceptions of external signs of poisoning, not because they might be true, but because the gap between outmoded, popular belief and modern, scientific fact could be turned to advantage. The medical jurist should note external appearances, he insisted, 'because the vulgar belief on the subject sometimes leads to such conduct or language on the part of the poisoner as betrays his secret at the time, and constitutes evidence of his guilt afterwards'.[41] Here Christison provides a salutary reminder that medico-legal testimony is in essential respects a matter of performance, an interaction between expert and popular knowledge. Although the modern expert should not himself countenance any trace of vulgar knowledge in his own work, a critical part of his skill lay in his capacity to effectively map scientific fact on to the broader and less stable network of public belief.

It is not difficult to understand why writers of toxicological texts would wish to reconfigure the interpretive space surrounding the poisoned body. Like the taming of poison's mythic history, subordinating external signs to analytically grounded indicators of poisoning emanating from the body's interior was of critical importance in demarcating a sphere of exclusive competence in which the toxicologist featured as the voice of expertise. Clearing away the accretions of the past served a further purpose. Freeing poison from the grip of the popular imagination, Christison insisted, had led to a more rational public response to cases of sudden death.[42] Commentators with no direct stake in a reconstituted toxicology voiced similar hopes. Macaulay contrasted the 'wild stories' of swelled tongues and discoloured bodies, which fanned public rumours of poison whenever an unexpected death was announced at the Stuart court, to the exemplary sobriety of his own times. Such tales ought to be preserved, he declared in true Whig fashion,

> for they furnish us with a measure of the intelligence and virtue of the generation which eagerly devoured them. That no rumour of the same kind has ever, in the present age, found credit among us . . . is to be attributed partly to the progress of medical and chemical science, but partly also, it may be hoped, to the progress which the nation has made in good sense, justice, and humanity.[43]

Taming poison's past, in this sense, served equally as an index of progress in knowledge and in morals. Yet toxicology's victory was neither

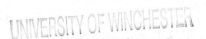

as clear-cut nor as complete as its professors would have wished. For a start, practitioners continued to indulge in unprofessional poison lore.[44] And removed from the confines of treatise literature, poison's imaginative resonances continued to fascinate the Victorian public, and to frustrate the modern toxicologist. A series of extended editorials appearing in the *London medical gazette* (a journal then under the editorship of Taylor), provides a stark indication of toxicology's fragile hold on the world of poison. Published in 1847, only a few months before the appearance of Taylor's *On poisons*, these editorials depict an expertise beset with difficulties generated from within and outside its own ranks.

It was in the first of these articles that the *Gazette* identified the rise of subtle, 'scientific' poisoning as the new threat facing society and its defenders.[45] It was in no doubt that this threat was real, and that men of science were in part responsible by promiscuously publicizing toxicological knowledge, capitalizing on the public interest in poison cases. Education, that vaunted engine of progress and civilization, was being perverted by a

> class of modern utilitarian philosophers who display their anxiety to establish a free trade in all descriptions of useful and useless knowledge, by doling out natural philosophy by the shilling's-worth, and by imparting a comprehensive insight into the mysteries of the occult sciences in lectures which are very considerately and judiciously limited to the brief period of half an hour.[46]

Despite the dismissive sarcasm, this represented a serious betrayal of Taylor's disciplinary aspirations. An unrestrained market in scientific knowledge, coupled with detailed newspaper reports of poison trials which at once alerted potential malefactors to the dangers of crude poisoning and provided information on how to refine their practices, threatened to undermine toxicology's capacity to contain the modern poisoner.

But it was neither indiscreet men of science nor journalists that came in for the heaviest criticism. The greater part of the *Gazette* series, in fact, was devoted to a critique of recent trends in contemporary literature. Within the past year, it complained, no less than three popular romances had appeared on the English market featuring the crimes of the Borgias. Such books, which it described as 'handbooks on poisoning', had made a direct impact. It was shortly after the appearance of several popular works on poison romances that the crime of poisoning assumed its new and fearful character, the *Gazette* lamented, 'which indicated that the wretches who employed this mode of assassination had become warned of the danger of detection that attends the administration of large quantities of any destructive drug, and had made themselves in some measure acquainted with the art of slow poisoning'.[47]

Without explicitly identifying the culprits, the *Gazette* detailed the crimes of these novelists. An unnamed 'lady writer' (Leticia Landon) had included in her final novel a case of prussic acid poisoning – fittingly, she had herself died shortly afterward of a medicinal overdose of that same substance. The malign influence of 'a certain French novel' (Alexander Dumas's *The Count of Monte Cristo*) came in for more sustained criticism as a stimulus to this dangerous revival. The article's centrepiece was a reprinted passage in which the Count contrasted the crude northern European poisoner with his more subtle Mediterranean counterpart. The former procures large doses of arsenic from local druggists, making futile attempts to disguise his criminal intentions, which only render him easier to detect. He proceeds to administer a dose, strong enough to kill an elephant, which is discoverable in 'whole spoonfuls' by the medical witness. 'But go beyond France, go to Aleppo, to Cairo, to Naples, or to Rome', the Count continues, 'and then you shall see passing in the street, fine tall upright men, fresh coloured and hearty, and you would never dream that *those men have been poisoned for three weeks, and will be quite dead in a month*'.[48] In the text of the novel itself, the passage that follows this one presents an even greater frustration to a modernized toxicological vision. Responding to his incredulous interlocutor who protested that such arts were lost to the modern poisoner, the Count observes: 'Come, come Madame, is anything ever lost to mankind? The arts and sciences travel around the world; things change their name, and ordinary people are deceived by it; the outcome is always the same'.[49]

But the *Gazette* reserved its most damning comment for a book by 'the most eloquent novelist of the day', a book amounting to 'a most complete revelation of the art of murder by poison, – a work which almost appears to have been written for the express purpose of reviving in the public mind an interest in the lost art of Italian poisoning'.[50] No one could be in any doubt that the culprit was Lytton's *Lucretia*, least of all Lytton himself, who promptly published a defence of his creation. In writing *Lucretia*, he protested, he had been careful not to give details that might lead to mischief:

the temporary success that attends the poisons employed by the murderers is made to depend solely on their selection of no drug to be procured by common-place villainy – in the secrets of chemical compounds, which at no shop could be purchased, of which no hint is conveyed, except that only by chemistry, the most erudite and skilful, they can possibly be combined. Rather than incur, however innocently, the possibility of supplying to one 'morbid idiosyncrasy' the agencies at the service of these modern Borgias, I have willingly invited the much more plausible accusation of far-fetched and impracticable devices, if ever existing, wholly lost to the invention, wholly out of the command, of guilt in the age in which we live.[51]

The *Gazette* was unimpressed. Reprinting copious passages from the offending text in a subsequent article, it castigated *Lucretia* not only for opening up the poison chest of the Borgias, reviving 'long slumbering' tales, but more dangerously for interweaving them with credible physiological realities that might be of use to 'the weak and the criminal'. In one scene, for example, Lucretia learns of a poison that is able to mimic angina pectoris, producing the appearance of muscular degeneration of the heart at autopsy. 'Can all these details be regarded merely as flights of innocent imagination,' the *Gazette* demanded: 'Are they not, on the contrary, lucid and substantial materials of instruction for the criminal, directly tending to enlarge his view of the subtlety and power of poisonous agents, and of the refined and baffling cautions which should be pursued for the purpose of accomplishing the extinction of human life, and of defeating justice'.[52]

Lytton's crime, then, was to offer a way of grafting the lure of ancient poison legend on to modern scientific knowledge, producing a deadly hybrid of science and the imagination. Malevolent readers might be stimulated by his depiction of slow poisoning to search out a credible scientific means of accomplishing this most coveted of the poisoner's dreams. The threat conjured by the *Gazette*, then, was one in which flights of past fancy were naturalized and made real by contemporary chemical knowledge. Belief in 'myths' like slow poison had obscured and impeded the path towards a properly scientific approach to the subject of poison. As a counter-measure, modern toxicology sought to marginalize myth, such that by mid-century the most up-to-date texts declined to engage in any form of non-scientific speculation. Yet, precisely at the time when poison lore had been purged, the *Gazette* warned, toxicologists found themselves faced with a new breed of slow poisoners, ones stripped of ancient myth, but employing scientific knowledge to reinvest poisoning with an aura of mystification. Despite its principled sobriety, then, mid-century toxicology had not succeeded in fully containing either poison's undisciplined past, or present.

In their efforts to construct a viable framework within which to deploy their proposed brand of expertise, toxicological writers had attempted, with only limited success, to draw a clear boundary around the historically and culturally embedded registers of poison. Yet, with Taylor's text serving as a model for a disciplined medico-legal approach to poison, toxicologists did have a sense of what their expertise ought to look like. The next chapter will consider the degree to which, at the level of toxicological practice, Taylor and his colleagues had succeeded in stripping out interferences of the imagination from their labours in the toxicological laboratory. But before entering into this domain, we need to consider a further disciplinary task facing the modern toxicologist: that of delineating not merely his proper domain of expertise, but the very object of his enquiries. What, in short, was a 'poison?'

This, perhaps surprisingly, was not a question that had been explicitly addressed in British textbooks prior to Taylor's 1848 treatise. Taylor, by contrast, set definition as the explicit aim of his opening chapter. To the popular mind, embodied in the courtroom by juries, judges, and advocates, the answer seemed obvious: 'A Poison is commonly defined to be a substance which, when administered in small quantity, is capable of acting deleteriously on the body'.[53] This definition, one that in Taylor's view had been too freely adopted by previous writers, traded on precisely what most captivated the public imagination about cases of poisoning – the asymmetrical process by which large and complex organisms succumbed to minute amounts of matter, reversing the clash of force by force which characterized traditional, physical modes of violence. This popular definition, however, fell quickly to the ground under toxicological scrutiny. Many of the substances most commonly recognized as poisons, he observes, were only lethal when administered in large doses, yet from a medico-legal point of view it was irrelevant whether death was caused, for example, by an ounce of nitre or a few grains of arsenic. Quantity, although compelling to a lay person, was no criterion for distinguishing between poison and other 'noxious things' which might be used for criminal purposes.

But abandoning the threshold of scale threatened to make toxicology look absurd from the vantage point of common sense. If substances were to be classed as poisons that only kill in large doses, then why not include common salt which, in large doses, acted like an irritant in much the same way as other substances routinely described as poisons? 'It may appear to be a violation of common language, to call the chloride of sodium a poison', Taylor admits, 'but assuredly it would be a greater inconsistency, to refuse to consider it as noxious, merely because it requires to be exhibited in a larger dose than some other irritants'.[54] One route out of this difficulty, Taylor proposes, might be to redefine poison not according to scale, but mode of introduction and action. A poison could then be defined as a substance which, 'taken internally, is capable of destroying life without acting mechanically on the system'.[55] Yet the internal/external boundary proves flawed, since a number of recognized poisons can act when applied to skin or to wounds. Without it, however, more confusion enters: if a poison can be a substance that is applied externally, then melted lead would have to be admitted as a poison, since it caused death when applied to the surface of a living body.

Another possibility – to admit internal and external routes for poison but to insist on the proviso of non-mechanical action – leads to a similar impasse. The stipulation about excluding mere mechanical action has a modern ring, in that it displaces the kind of crude physicalism exemplified by Mead in the previous century, and keeps substances like ingested pins and ground glass (a favourite topic of ancient authorities) happily outside the class of poisons. But what about the case of boiling liquids? Is their action purely mechanical? If not, then they are poisons. If so, then mineral acids and alkalis, which according to Taylor act in an identical fashion, could not be classed as poisons. 'These remarks', Taylor concludes, 'show that it is, indeed, very difficult to comprise in a few words an accurate description of what should be understood by the term "poison"'.[56]

In the face of this definitional conundrum, Taylor's advice to medical witnesses was primarily one of caution – to be on their guard against basing their testimony on facile and arbitrary boundaries relying on dosage or action. But the difficulties posed by the lack of a clear referent for the subject matter of toxicology extended beyond the circumstances of individual cases, raising more fundamental questions about how to address the problem of poison at a social and a legislative level. Nowhere is this more apparent than when toxicologists and others were faced with a question debated since classical times: what was the difference between a poison and a medicine?

The double meaning of *pharmakon* and *venenum*, a topic singled out by Jacques Derrida, most notably, as an exemplary instance of the contingent origins of our seemingly natural categories of linguistic and conceptual order, was recognized by ancient and early-modern commentators as an inherent feature of discussions both of poison and of medicine.[57] Pliny, in his *Natural history*, used *venenum* interchangeably as remedy and poison. The celebrated Roman jurist Gaius, observing that the word 'is neutral in meaning and includes not only that which kills but that which cures as well,' insisted that anyone using the term 'must add whether it is beneficial or harmful'.[58] The sixteenth century iatro-chemical reformer Paracelsus famously declared that 'all things are poison and nothing is without poison', using this insight to denounce the medical establishment as monopolistic incompetents. Early-modern English practitioners similarly pondered the porous boundary between poison and medicine. Culpeper and his colleagues agreed with ancient and contemporary authors who described certain types of medicines – purgatives, for example – as poisons:

> For the understanding of this: Observe first, that Galen used the word deadly for that which may kil, or that which may do good sometimes, though it may kil by accident. Note secondly, that some Medicines always hurt, and never do good; these are poisons, and so must be called. But they which sometimes do hurt, are not to be accounted poisons, and they which sometimes do good, are not to be excluded from the number of poisons.[59]

Medical and popular dictionaries and encyclopedias from the eighteenth and early nineteenth centuries continued to stress this overlap in their entries on poisons, an association that was made increasingly apparent by contemporary developments in experimental pharmacology and physiology predicated on the poison–medicine continuum.[60]

It would have come as no real surprise to his readers, then, that in seeking out a workable definition for poison, Taylor remarked on its proximity to medicine: 'No one can draw a definite boundary between a poison and a medicine', he observed in the preface to his second edition. 'The greater number of poisons are useful medicines when properly employed, and nearly every substance in the catalogue of medicines may be converted into an instrument of death if improperly administered'.[61] Yet however obvious it might be as a matter of fact, the porous boundary between poison and medicine was a source of considerable difficulty. Given the overall aim of his book – that of laying the medico-legal foundations for resisting the rising tide of criminal poisoning – Taylor required a definition of poison that would enable anything that fell within its scope to be subjected to functioning regimes of containment. Taylor was seeking, in other words, to give poison a substantive, categorical existence with clearly demarcated borders capable of being patrolled. In this light, the fact that under most definitional schemas 'the whole class of medicines' would fall into the category of poisons, made the task of constructing poison as a stable regulatory object deeply problematic.[62]

Nowhere can this be better illustrated than through the convoluted contemporary attempts to control what by mid-century had come to be known as 'the poison trade'. The 1840s and 1850s are well known as the key decades in the longstanding campaign to reform the English medical profession. Legislative proposals were tabled on a near yearly basis aimed at reforming the medical licensing and educational system, and providing the public with a clear set of distinctions between 'regular' and 'quack' practitioners. Within this campaign there were several (often shifting) lines of demarcation. Reform-minded champions of scientifically trained general practitioners like Thomas Wakley criticized both the entrenched corporate elite and the welter of 'untrained' practitioners masquerading as medical advisers to the people. This latter category included not only notorious figures like the 'hygiest' James Morison and the medical botanist Isaac Coffin – both targets of the *Lancet*'s 'Anti-Quackery Society' – but also 'ignorant' chemists and druggists who for decades, from the perspective of the beleaguered general practitioner, had been encroaching on his professional territory by dispensing not merely medicinal preparations but also advice, with many even undertaking home consultations.

In one formulation, then, chemists and druggists were lumped together with quacks as threats to public well-being, the *Lancet* claiming, for example, that 'the deaths which are likely to occur from the ill-treatment of the sick by quacks and prescribing druggists, throw into shadow all the murders and all the deaths from violence that could happen to any state of society, the murders of war being excepted'.[63] Yet having yoked prescribing druggists to the vile ranks of quackery, the editorial offered a further level of differentiation: 'The great mass of chemists and druggists in England receive no professional education; they are ignorant of the scientific parts of chemistry, and they have no general acquaintance with pharmacy'.[64]

If, as this particular *Lancet* editorial seemed to suggest, the general practitioners' criticism of chemists and druggists was restricted to those without 'professional education', then they would find a staunch set of allies from within a distinct sector of the drug trade – amongst the ranks of 'pure' pharmacy. The term 'chemist and druggist', as S. W. F. Holloway has shown, covered a vast range of activities and personnel: from the oil-man and general grocer selling preparations as part of a general retail trade, to the pharmaceutical specialist.[65] From the vantage point of the latter, who from 1841 were represented by the Pharmaceutical Society, the *Lancet*'s identification of 'ignorance' was the salient point of demarcation between those who should be considered inside and outside the medical pale. Established by Jacob Bell and several other metropolitan chemists, the Pharmaceutical Society, through its in-house organ (the *Pharmaceutical journal*) and its vigorous parliamentary lobbying activities, waged a sustained campaign for a legislative framework that would distinguish 'pharmacy' as a scientific profession from untrained, and thus unlicensed, tradespeople.

The Pharmaceutical Society's emphasis on knowledge as the sole legitimate ground for a monopoly of practice, dovetailed perfectly with the ethos of professionalizing reform advocated by champions of the general practitioner, and it is therefore not surprising that the two groups were able to find common ground. Thus, as Peter Bartrip has observed, the Provincial Medical and Surgical Association (the forerunner of the modern BMA) and the Pharmaceutical Society worked closely together on legislative change, a partnership that culminated in the Arsenic Act of 1851.[66] The regulation of the sale of poison, in particular the sale of poisons used in medicinal preparations, was in fact central to both medical and pharmaceutical reform. For the general practitioner, achieving a monopoly on prescribing medicinal poisons would drive quacks out of business. From the point of view of Bell's pharmacists, restricting the sale of such items to those who had passed the Society's qualifying examination would be symbolic of a public trust conferred upon them as practitioners of recognized skill and discretion, and would go a long way to blunt contemporary criticisms appearing in the lay and medical press which denounced chemists as 'venal poison mongers',[67] whose indiscriminate sale of deadly substances swelled the numbers of accidental poisonings, and abetted the designs of murderous criminals.

Proposals for restricting the poison trade, however, were not confined to the educational tests favoured by Bell and his colleagues. Instead, in response to widespread public criticism of lax and ignorant dispensing practices, the legislative formula most often proposed for dealing with the problem centred on placing restrictive conditions on their sale. Proposals of this kind were numerous: establishing a poison register which would record the details of each purchase of a poisonous agent; requiring a letter of authorization for the purchase of small amounts of poison; mandating the use of special shaped and coloured bottles boldly labelled 'POISON' for the use of compounds containing poisonous material; constructing separate 'poison closets' in chemists' shops to be kept under lock and key, and entered by the chemist with due solemnity and caution, for example.

These sorts of measures, from the perspective of the *Pharmaceutical journal*, would be at once ineffectual, dangerous, and a threat to commerce. Compared with their continental counterparts, for whom a restricted medical market was an accepted fact of life, English men and women, Jacob Bell argued, were 'much more addicted to taking physic',[68] and therefore would not, 'for the sake of any theoretic notions of perfection, be debarred from the enjoyment of things which custom has rendered necessary'.[69] Registers and letters of authorization, he insisted, would be seen by the public as a violation of its long-standing 'right' to self-medication. 'Poison closets' were equally abhorred. They would, in the first place, merely add to the public's resentment of un-English infringements of medical liberty, customers waiting for their routine cordials being thus turned into 'applicants at a *bureau de police*'.[70]

More problematically, the construction of such cordoned-off spaces in every chemist shop threatened to revisit the difficult subject raised by toxicologists like Taylor in their quest for a working definition of poison: how was poison to be distinguished from medicine? Poison closets, their critics feared, would translate this conundrum into stark, spatial terms. 'The relative size of the closet and the shop does not appear to enter into the calculation,' the *Pharmaceutical journal* observed, 'although it would be found if the experiment were tried, that the shop would be little more than a closet, and the poison department about the size of an ordinary shop'. Regulationists would do well to 'consider what must be the feelings of patients on seeing the dispenser every two or three minutes unlock the ponderous door and enter the poison chamber to fetch each dose of calomel, laudanum, or other medicines ordered in their prescriptions'.[71] Plans to label items as 'poison' would cause similar alarm, interfering with the public's faith in and willingness to follow doctors' advice. Since 'nine out of ten of the substances which we sell are poisons', Bell warned a parliamentary committee of inquiry, any labelling scheme would cast a pall over the whole therapeutic enterprise: 'A man sees a large label, with the word 'poison' upon it; he will not touch it, and he goes to his doctor and says, "You are giving me poison"'.[72]

The problem for the pharmacist, then, was that such restrictions on dispensing, by rendering transparent just how many of the everyday compounds applied for by the public were classifiable as poison, would alarm and potentially alienate his client base. For medical practitioners, segregation and labelling were equally troublesome, particularly at mid-century. As Logie Barrow and others have shown, alternative medical systems were flourishing precisely at this time, galvanized in large part by the aggressive professionalizing claims of orthodox medical reformers.[73] Many of these medical 'sectarians' grounded their criticism of regular practitioners ('allopaths') by pointing to the myriad of toxic substances which they employed. Orthodox medicine, they charged, was literally poisoning its patients. Isaac Coffin, the founder of medical botany in Britain, was particularly insistent on this point. In the inaugural issue of his proselytizing *Botanical journal and medical reformer*, he set the tone for his long and bitter struggle against medical orthodoxy, inveighing against 'mineral loving, and *poison* dealing doctors'.[74] Poisonous medicines, he insisted in a later issue, were the 'principal cause' of increased sickness amongst the populace. Coffinism, in turn, represented the remedy for 'the poisonous practices pursued by the faculty'.[75]

Another thorn in the side of medical regulars, the quintessential exponent of 'quackery' James Morison, similarly inveighed against medicinal poisons, not merely in the printed word but in several of his widely circulated lithographs used to advertise his 'British College of Health'. The best known of these images contrasts two 'medical trees,' a diseased one growing next to a shop, pointedly named 'The Lancet and Co.', which displayed bottles of prussic acid, laudanum, mercury and arsenic in its window, and one flourishing in the shadow of Morison's college. A second tableau made the links between regular medicine and the contemporary scourge of poisoning even more strikingly. It features a queue of customers formed inside a chemist's shop, each seeking to purchase poisons. Amidst ignorant self-medicators and poisoning doctors were characters drawn from the annals of criminal poisoning: assassins from the Stuart court, the Marchioness de Brinvilliers, Madame Lafarge, and even Lytton's Lucretia, converse whilst waiting patiently to be served – fully confident that their nefarious needs will be met. The difference between the doctors who use poison in their practice, and the professed criminal poisoners, the poster's caption noted, 'is only a question of a few GRAINS or DROPS'.[76]

Medical sectarians like Coffin and Morison thus traded directly on the image of an orthodox medicine deeply implicated in the numerous social ills stemming from the trade in poisons. Many regular practitioners, moreover, acknowledged the force of the criticism, and, as a feature of the broader push for professional reform, pressure was increasingly brought to bear for the adoption of a more restrained approach to medication. A *Lancet* correspondent, complaining of the routine therapeutic recourse to 'poisons' like mercury, insisted that such practices amounted to a dangerous form of quackery: 'In every town in England, the number of constitutions ruined, and delicate persons murdered ... all produced by mercury, marks the wretched, indiscriminate and empirical abuse of this powerful [poison] in common practice'.[77] From within the ranks of reform-minded practitioners, then, the poison-medicine continuum could serve as the ground of inter- and intra-professional conflict. In this fraught context, any legislative measures drawing attention to the problem would, they feared, do little to promote a judicious resolution.

Poison's place within the contested world of medical and pharmaceutical reform, however unsettling, could not be ignored. The dangers of the free trade in poison, and its connections to the epidemic of criminal poisoning that seemed to be ravaging Victorian Britain, were loudly denounced in a public press that demanded a solution. Reform-minded bodies responded by seeking to reconcile public concern with their own professional considerations. The first tangible fruit of this effort was the 1851 Arsenic Act.

The 1851 act, which placed the sale of arsenic, unlike other poisons, under a series of restrictive measures, ensured that the elusive category 'poison' had at least one legally sanctioned constitutive element. It aimed to restrict sales to adults either personally known to the vendor, or in the presence of a witness known to both parties. The details of each transaction had to be recorded in a poison register, and if the quantity purchased were less than ten pounds in weight, the arsenic was to be mixed with soot or indigo for easier recognition on the part of a potential poisoning victim. In many respects, arsenic was an obvious candidate for isolation, as the nation's first poison to be recognized in law. It clearly conformed to the public image of a dangerous poison: it was fatal in minute doses (between two and four grains, according to most authorities);[78] it was colourless and odourless, and thus easy to administer by stealth; and, most importantly, it had been the agent of choice in the vast majority of criminal cases that had been splashed across the pages of the lay and medical press in recent decades.[79] From a toxicological point of view, arsenic also stood as a useful archetype for poison. By far the most discussed poison in all the modern medico-legal treatises, it was at once highly toxic and comparatively easy to trace, with Christison claiming that there were 'few substances in nature, and perhaps hardly any other poison, whose presence can be detected in such minute quantities and with so great certainty'.[80]

Arsenic, synonymous both with the perils of unregulated poison and with the promise of its scientific resolution, thus seemed an appropriate anchoring point for the legal and scientific management of the poison problem. But, according to leading toxicological commentators, the Arsenic Act in practice was something of a disappointment. Enforcement of its provisions, for one thing, proved weak, and, before long, regulationists were complaining that the 'free trade' in poison was as robust as ever. It was, Taylor complained, little more than a decade after its passage, 'a dead letter, so far as the public safety is concerned'.[81] Conceptually too, the isolation of arsenic as an indisputable 'poison' was problematic. Even promoters of the act acknowledged that there was no principled justification for isolating arsenic as the sole legislative referent for the ambiguous term 'poison'. In a pamphlet circulated to all MPs prior to the vote on the 1851 Arsenic Bill, the Provincial Medical and Surgical Association's spokesman on poison reform explained that the Association 'thought it desirable to attack the GREAT ARSENIC EVIL first, leaving the important subject of the sale of poisonous drugs for a future opportunity; for it is far better to aim at the destruction of one prominent enemy, than to weaken our forces by attempting to combat many'.[82] The *Pharmaceutical journal*, in voicing qualified support for the measure at this early stage, elaborated on the pragmatic arguments for isolating arsenic. The PMSA, it thought, had restricted its proposals to arsenic 'fearing that a general denunciation of poisons would be met by the *argumentum ad absurdum*, on the ground that almost all medicines would come under the definition'.[83]

The act's arbitrary classification, the *Pharmaceutical journal* was suggesting, was necessary in order to prevent all medicines from being treated – and viewed by the public – as poisons. In this sense, arsenic was a convenient focal point, allowing the vexed problem of definition to be avoided in the name of expediency. Yet the ostensible stability of arsenic as a substantive poison belied a more complicated reality. Like other 'strong poisons', arsenic had a staggering range of applications in the Victorian world. The key ingredient in one of the leading patent medicines of the day ('Fowler's Solution'), arsenic was used to combat skin disorders, cancers and fevers. In Victorian homes it was used as a vermin killer, and as a dye in paint, fabrics and wallpapers. Arsenic could be found in the candles that lit these homes, in certain types of cooking utensil, and in the sweets consumed by their inhabitants.[84] Its agricultural uses included anti-parasitical dips for sheep and anti-fungal preparations for grain.

Arsenic's dual existence, as an article of everyday life and as an instrument for the criminal assault on life, was a tension that had to be lived with. But even the bedrock assumption about arsenic – that if ingested in a small but well-defined quantity, it would prove universally fatal – was called into question shortly after the passage of the Arsenic Act. The source of this qualification, moreover, threatened to undermine the larger process of 'disciplining' poison that has been the focus of this chapter. It is fitting, then, to conclude with a return to the realm of fable, a purported discovery from a most unlikely source that seemed to question arsenic's position as the cornerstone of the legal and scientific model of containment. At the centre of this controversy stood a community of amorous and robust Austrian peasants who habitually medicated themselves with copious doses of arsenic.

It was *The chemist*, a normally rather dry, technical journal, which first broke the fabulous news from the region of Styria, a mountainous enclave on the Austro-Hungarian border. In 1854, the journal publicized a series of letters that had lately been making the rounds in continental medical journals.[85] The letters were penned by the Swiss naturalist Johann Jakob von Tschudi. Until then best known for his tales of wonder from the South American jungle, von Tschudi's return to Europe, commentators ruefully observed, had not dimmed his enthusiasm for the exotic. Instead, his letters announced the discovery of habitual arsenic eating amongst the Stryian peasantry. These 'toxicophagi' (or 'poison eaters') had two aims: to procure a 'fresh and healthy appearance,' and to improve their 'wind' – that is, their respiratory capabilities. In both cases the Styrians met with success. 'Young toxicophagi', von Tschudi admiringly observed, 'are distinguished by the freshness of their complexion and by the aspect of flourishing health'. As for their wind, the arsenic eaters 'ascend without difficulty heights which would have been almost insurmountable without this practice'. Their method of arsenic eating was to start with small doses, about half a grain, which they consumed morning and night for a long period until their bodies become habituated. They then increased the dose incrementally until they attained the desired effect. Four grains a day, a quantity at the upper end of the 'poison' threshold set by English experts, was not an uncommon level to achieve.[86]

Before long the Styrian peasants were beginning to exercise the English toxicological world. The idea that human bodies could tolerate, and even benefit from self-prescribed fatal doses of the nation's most notorious poison flew in the face of both professional knowledge and the legislative framework so recently and painstakingly constructed around the poison trade. Not surprisingly, it drew a derisory response from leading toxicologists – it was, according to Taylor, founded on 'absurd and exaggerated statements . . . utterly inconsistent with all that is known concerning the action of arsenic'.[87] Outright dismissal proved insufficient to quash the reports, however, and accounts circulating in the popular press provoked the *Association medical journal* (successor to the *PMSJ* as the official voice of the PMSA) to run a series of articles in the summer of 1856 dedicated to a thorough debunking of the story.

The timing of the articles was not accidental. Several high-profile poisoning trials had recently concluded, involving cases of suspected secret poisoning, one of which concerned a charge of wife poisoning against Joseph Wooler. Jane Wooler had died in June 1855, following a long and mysterious illness anxiously watched over by her medical attendants and her loving husband, a retired 'mercantile gentleman' who, in his professional travels to distant lands, had accumulated a large stock of poisonous medicines which he admitted using on both himself and his wife. As her condition deteriorated, her doctors began to suspect that she was suffering from an extended exposure to small amounts of arsenic, and, following her death, toxicologists of the first rank, including Taylor and Christison, were consulted. Tests confirmed the presence of arsenical traces, and Wooler was brought to trial in December.

The case itself ended in an acquittal, but remained a topic of debate, with a host of theories about the cause of Mrs Wooler's demise being proposed in the lay and medical press. The most striking – and most irritating to the toxicologists involved – was the widely circulated suggestion that Mrs Wooler was an English arsenic eater. Reviewing his own participation in this 'remarkable' case for the *Edinburgh medical journal*, Christison poured scorn on this suggestion. Nevertheless, he continued, such claims, 'so dangerous if false, so revolutionary if true', demanded serious rebuttal. As far as the particulars of the Wooler case went, the facts pointed away from a Styrian connection. Mrs Wooler, Christison insisted, was in the first instance 'too amiable and right-thinking a woman to perpetrate such an act of folly'. Furthermore, von Tschudi's reports had come to popular attention too recently for her to have become a dedicated arsenic eater. From a more general, medical viewpoint, Christison was confident that experienced medical men would treat the tale as 'pure fable'. While acknowledging the use of arsenic by physicians to treat certain chronic conditions, experience had shown that 'the human body, instead of becoming habituated to these doses, as in the case of opium, tobacco, and some other vegetable poisons, acquires, in reality, a greater, and not a less, sensitiveness to its action'. If it were von Tschudi's intent to overturn this conventional wisdom, the onus was on him to submit 'proof proportioned to its improbability'. Instead, his reports contained no first-hand observation and experiment, and thus ought not to be entertained, either in an English courtroom or in the English medico-legal canon.[88]

These concerns provided the primary focus for the *AMJ* series on arsenic-eating in the summer of 1856. Its author, the surgeon W. B. Kesteven, made clear that his purpose was to neutralize the possibly damaging impact of the report upon the conduct of criminal trials. Accordingly, Kesteven adopted a predominantly legalistic frame for his discussion. His first instalment provided the full text of von Tschudi's account, prefacing it with the cautionary remark that 'in a medico-legal point of view, which is that from which this subject must be regarded as having more especially called for investigation, . . . it will be shown to be useless as a means of defence in criminal proceedings'. In the second article, Kesteven focused on the dubious modes of transmission through which the Styrian legend had become a matter of public knowledge. It directed particular scorn at the ostensibly scientific account in F. W. Johnston's *Chemistry of common life*. Johnston, a Durham chemist and fellow of the Royal Society, had devoted a chapter of his book, serialized in *Blackwood's Edinburgh magazine*, to poison-eaters.[89] In it he reported on the Styrian romance, crediting it as a matter of fact and embellishing it as a singular route to domestic harmony: 'Thus even cruel arsenic, so often the minister of crime and the parent of sorrow, bears a blessed jewel in its forehead; and, as a love-awakener, becomes . . . the harbinger of happiness, the soother of ardent longings, the bestower of contentment and peace'!'[90]

In criticizing Johnston's account, Kesteven worried about its effect on the credulous reader, but again his main focus was on the credulous courtroom. If 'such marvellous statements appear, invested with all the prestige and authority of science,' he demanded, 'can we be surprised if the poisoner shall seek to screen himself behind seemingly authentic and unanswerable statements of the innocuousness of the agent he has employed, and which chemical analysis has demonstrated beyond possibility of his denial'?[91] Here Kesteven expressed frustration at the artful possibilities of subverting hard toxicological demonstration. The Styrian myth threatened to detach questions of proof from what for him were the stable grounds of chemistry, and to place them in the realm of fiction. Accordingly, in his final article, Kesteven subjected the tale to the twin rigours of scientific and legal scrutiny. Von Tschudi's report lacked all the

hallmarks of evidentiary admissibility: no analysis of the substance purported to be arsenic had been made, no eyewitness accounts of dosing
had been brought forward, and no information derived from a systematic
study of Styrian mortality returns had been gathered. He then reported
on his own attempts to generate such a body of evidence. He had circulated a questionnaire to all those who pretended direct knowledge of the
practice, enquiring as to the foundations of their claims. None were satisfactory, in his view. They were, adopting the quasi-legalistic discourse
appropriate to his main object of concern, devoid of 'direct personal
testimony', 'simply hearsay evidence'. 'It is hoped', he concludes, that as a
result of his labours, courts will refuse to 'admit inferences from such
unsupported statements, as having the same weight and value as those
drawn from indisputable fact'.[92]

Yet, contrary to expectation, and certainly to Kesteven's hopes, the
legend did not die. In the courtroom, it gained an even greater notoriety
some two years following the Wooler trial when, during the sensational
Scottish trial of Madeline Smith, the Styrian approach to health and
beauty was invoked by the defence to explain Smith's possession of copious amounts of arsenic. In the subsequent decade, moreover, the medical
and pharmaceutical press carried reports indicating that Kesteven's
demand for the production of 'hard evidence' had been taken up, with
surprising results. In 1860, the eminent chemist Henry Roscoe delivered
a paper before the Manchester Literary and Philosophical Society, in
which he claimed to have received six grams of a white substance forwarded by a colleague in Graz, accompanied by a certificate from a
Styrian district judge testifying to its local origin. Careful analysis, Roscoe
reported, showed that the substance was pure arsenious acid, and he
concluded that arsenic was both well known and widely distributed in
Styria, and was taken regularly 'in quantities supposed sufficient to produce immediate death'.[93] Others supported Roscoe's claim, and in 1864
the *Edinburgh medical journal* published a communication by Dr Craig
Maclagan which provided the fullest and best documented account to
date – a set of lengthy case studies conducted personally by him which
contained all the technologies of proof demanded by Kesteven. Previous
dismissals of the Styrian reports as 'pure fable', though warranted at the
time, were in Maclagan's view 'no longer tenable'.[94]

The reasons for the intense irritation provoked by Styrian arsenic-
eating are embedded in the topics covered in this chapter. Simply put, it
disrupted the interlocking containment efforts of toxicological modernizers. It testified to the continuing power of poison 'myth' at mid-century,

challenging definitional regimes and the legislative arrangements that followed from them. It posed a further disruption, by calling attention to the core practical and symbolic order of toxicological proof. In a case of criminal poisoning, such proof was predicated on viewing poisons like arsenic as foreign substances – matter out of place – in an otherwise normal body. By suggesting that bodies coming before the toxicologist could in themselves be less than pure, the Styrian story served as a stark indicator of the difficulties entailed not only in detecting cases of genuine criminal administration, but of justifying these findings in court. The problems of toxicological proof, at both the symbolic and practical levels, are the subject of the following chapter.

Notes

1 For a comparative history of the rise of medical jurisprudence, see Erwin Ackerknecht, 'Early history of legal medicine'; 'Legal medicine in transition'; and 'Legal medicine becomes a modern science' in *Cyba symposia* 11 (1950–51), pp. 1286–9, pp. 1290–8, pp. 1299–304. For discussions in the English context, see, in addition to my *Bodies of evidence: medicine and the politics of the English inquest, 1830–1926* (Baltimore and Johns Hopkins University Press), Michael Clark and Catherine Crawford (eds), *Legal medicine in history* (Cambridge: Cambridge University Press, 1994); Catherine Crawford, 'A scientific profession: medical reform and forensic medicine in British periodicals of the early nineteenth century', in Roger French and Andrew Wear (eds), *British medicine in an age of reform* (London: Routledge, 1991), pp. 203–30; and Jennifer Ward, 'Origins and development of forensic medicine and forensic science in England, 1823–1946', Ph.D. dissertation, Open University, 1993. For Scottish legal medicine, see Anne Crowther and Brenda White, *On soul and conscience: the medical expert and crime* (Aberdeen: Aberdeen University Press, 1988).

2 Crowther and White, *On soul and conscience* ch. 1; Crowther, 'The toxicology of Robert Christison: European influences and British practice in the early nineteenth century', in José Ramón Bertomeu-Sánchez and Agustí Nieto-Galan (eds), *Chemistry, medicine and crime: Orfila and his times* (New York: Science History Publications, 2006). The information in this and the following paragraph is drawn largely from these sources.

3 Christison was made assistant editor of the *Edinburgh medical and surgical journal* in 1820, and joint editor in 1827 a position he held until 1832. *Edinburgh medical journal* 17 (1905), 4, cited in Crowther, 'The toxicology'.

4 The best institutional account of the early years of English forensic medicine in J. Ward, 'The rise', ch. 2.

5 See Burney, *Bodies of evidence*, and Crawford, 'A scientific profession'. 'The

sure, the unerring test of the state of professional knowledge in any nation, is the character of the medical testimony in its forensic investigations', the *Lancet* ventured in 1832, adding that, in its current form, this test had 'mortifying' results for native practice. 'Forensic medicine as a test of knowledge', *Lancet* 1 (1831–32), pp. 621–2, p. 621.

6   In 1836 the Royal College of Physicians added medical jurisprudence to its list of required – although again not examinable – courses. By 1840, the Royal College of Surgeons had followed suit. These developments came too late for Smith, who had resigned his chair in November 1830, amidst internal university recriminations including accusations of madness; after a brief editorship of *London medical repository*, Smith entered a debtors' prison, where he died fifteen months later.

7   The *Lancet* seized on these features in denouncing the LSA regulations as a 'barefaced and unqualified practice of extortion'. 'Dr Thompson and his benefactors', *Lancet* 2 (1830–1), pp. 690–4, p. 691. It was not until the late 1850s that the LSA required an examination in medical jurisprudence and toxicology.

8   Among them were the public-health activists Thomas Southwood Smith and Hector Gavin, and the statistician William Guy.

9   Taylor (1806–80) studied chemistry as well as medicine at Guy's, and developed an interest in medical jurisprudence there and on several visits to Paris. In addition to his professorship of medical jurisprudence (which he held until 1878), Taylor was appointed joint lecturer on chemistry in 1832, becoming sole lecturer in 1851. He was elected FRS in 1845, MRCP in 1848, FRCP in 1853, and was awarded an honorary MD from St Andrews in 1852. His practice as a toxicological expert in both criminal and civil cases – his principal source of income – was successful enough to leave him with an estate of £60,000 at his death. For more on Taylor, in addition to the *New dictionary of national biography*, see Noel Coley, 'Alfred Swaine Taylor, MD, FRS (1806–80): forensic toxicologist', *Medical history* 35 (1991), pp. 409–27.

10   See Ward, 'Origins and development', ch. 2.

11   On the public standing of chemistry at the opening of the nineteenth century, see Jan Golinski, *Science as public culture: chemistry and enlightenment in Britain, 1760–1820* (Cambridge: Cambridge University Press, 1992).

12   Robert Christison, 'On the present state of medical evidence', *Edinburgh medical review* 23 (n.s.) (1851), pp. 401–30, p. 402.

13   Robert Christison, *A treatise on poisons* (Edinburgh: Adam Black, 1829).

14   Alfred Swaine Taylor, *On poisons in relation to medical jurisprudence* (London: John Churchill, 1848). It is notable that Taylor included a limited discussion of this experimental literature on practical grounds alone: in a then-recent case of opium poisoning, a medical witness was examined by court as to the mode of death caused by the drug. 'This', he observed, 'is sufficient to justify the introduction of a few remarks on the subject in this place'. (*Ibid.*, p. 16)

15 Even in cases of 'special difficulty', when more obviously 'expert' witnesses were sought out, they appeared not as official adjuncts of the prosecution but as independent advisers, who might equally have acted on behalf of the defence. In practice, however, experts like Taylor appeared almost exclusively for the prosecution in criminal cases. It was not until the 1880s that official Home Office analysts were named, and even then these appointees were nominally independent, nominated by the medical colleges, and free to appear on either side of a case. See Ward, 'Origins and development', ch. 4, and Burney, *Bodies of evidence*, especially. ch. 4.

16 Taylor, *On poisons* (1848), p. v. This sense of pressing practical need, and the humiliation that would follow from a failed courtroom appearance by an unprepared practitioner, was routinely invoked by lecturers and writers on medical jurisprudence as an incentive for students to attend their courses and buy their texts.

17 As Katherine Watson has found, by the early 1840s an informal network of individuals scattered over the country was beginning to emerge as recognized poison specialists, who might be consulted by coroners and by the Home Office in cases of 'special difficulty'. According to Watson's count, Taylor, as the only figure with a genuine national reach, appeared most frequently (thirty-one cases between 1844 and 1869), followed by the Bristol-based William Herapath (twenty-two cases between 1834 and 1867). Katherine Watson *Poisoned lives: English poisoners and their victims* (London and New York: London and Hambeldon, 2004), p. 167.

18 Robert Hooper, *A compendious medical dictionary. Containing an explanation of the terms in anatomy, physiology, surgery, materia medica, chemistry, and practice of physic* (London: Murray and Highley, 1799), 'Toxicology' entry.

19 Robert Hooper, *Lexicon medicum, or medical dictionary* (London: Longmans, Hurst, Rees, Orme and Co., 1820), 'Toxicology'. The earliest literary use of the word I have found is in Thomas Love Peacock's satirical Gothic tale *Crotchet castle* (1831), in which 'Mr Henbane, the toxicologist' indulges in animal experiments in an attempt to discover a universal antidote to poison, and is ultimately poisoned by his antidote.

20 John Forbes, Alexander Tweedie and John Conolly, *Cyclopaedia of practical medicine*, 4 vols (London: Sherwood, Gilbert and Piper, 1833–34), 4, p. 167.

21 Favourite topics included the workings of amulets and charms providing a universal safeguard against poison (serpent or unicorn horns; gems that gleamed or glass that shattered in the presence of poison), and the myriad of ways in which poison might enter the body (e.g. by sight or hearing).

22 Lyn Thorndike, *A history of magic and experimental science*, 8 vols (London and New York: Macmillan, 1923–58), 3, p. 525.

23 Clyde Pharr, 'The interdiction of magic in Roman law', *Transactions and proceedings of the American philological association* 63 (1932), pp. 269–95.

24 Thorndike, *History of magic* 2, p. 904; Pharr, 'The interdiction of magic', p. 286.

25 Ireland, 'Chaucer's toxicology', p. 77.

26 Thomas Spratt, cited in J. A. Paris and J. S. M. Fonblanque, *Medical jurisprudence*, 3 vols (London: W. Phillips, 1823), 2, p. 137.

27 William Ramesey, *Lifes* [*sic*] *security, or, a phylosophical and physical discourse shewing the names, natures, & vertues of all sorts of venomes and venemous things, as in poysons in general and in particular* (London, 1665), p. 11. Ramesey is listed in a number of nineteenth-century toxicological bibliographies as the author of the first poison treatise in vernacular English, e.g. Forbes's *Cyclopaedia* 4, p. 167, and James Copland, *Dictionary of practical medicine* (London: Longman, Brown, Green, and Longmans, 1858), p. 439. A few years later, in their *Sixth book of practical physick: of occult or hidden diseases* (London: Peter Cole, 1662), the physicians Daniel Sennert, Nicholas Culpeper, and Abdiah Cole also cast doubt on the claim that, in the natural realm, 'the same poyson should kill sometimes sooner, sometimes later' (p. 31). However, they admitted the possibility that this may be true in cases involving witchcraft, incantation, and charms (see bk 4, ch. 2, 'What inchantments, poysonous witchcraft, and magick are', pp. 86–8).

28 Richard Mead, *A mechanical account of poisons in several essays* (London: Ralph Smith, 1702), pp. 111–12. For a discussion of early modern theories of poison's action, see M. P. Earles, 'Early theories of the mode of action of drugs and poisons', *Annals of science* 17:2 (1961), pp. 97–110, and M. P. Earles, 'Experiments with drugs and poisons in the 17th and 18th centuries', in *Annals of science* 19:4 (1963), pp. 241–54. It should be noted that this naturalistic turn dovetails with discussions more directly concerned with witchcraft: Reginald Scot's scepticism about the reality of witchcraft, for example, led him to argue that much of what passed as acts of witchcraft were in reality cases of undetected poisonings. See Keith Thomas, *Religion and the decline of magic* (New York: Charles Scribner's Sons, 1971), p. 645.

29 G. E. Male, *An epitome of juridical or forensic medicine* (London: T. and G. Underwood, 1816), p. 14.

30 G. E. Male, *Elements of juridical or forensic medicine*, 2nd edn (London: E. Cox and Son, 1818), p. 23. Emphasis added.

31 Paris and Fonblanque, *Medical jurisprudence* 2, pp. 132, p. 138. Emphasis original.

32 Christison, *A treatise*, pp. 30, 31.

33 George Eglisham, *The forerunner of revenge* (London, 1642, orig. 1626), pp. 10–11. For Eglisham, see David Harley, 'Political post-mortems and morbid anatomy in seventeenth-century England', *Social history of medicine* 7 (1994), pp. 1–28; for a discussion of the controversy, and poisoning in the Stuart court more generally, see Alastair Bellany, *Politics of court scandal in early modern England* (Cambridge University Press, 2002).

34 Sennert *et al.*, *Sixth book*, p. 33.
35 Malcolm Gaskell, 'Reporting murder: fiction in the archives in early modern England', *Social history* 23:1 (1998), pp. 1–30, pp. 22–3.
36 'Trial of Mr Angus', *Edinburgh medical and surgical journal* 5 (1809), pp. 220–9, p. 226; *The Times* (15 August 1816), p. 3.
37 *The Times* (27 March 1848), p. 7.
38 Male, *An epitome* (1816), p. 34; Paris and Fonblanque, *Medical jurisprudence* 2, p. 182. Juvenal described the victims' 'blackened' corpses in the first of his *Satires*.
39 Christison, *A treatise*, pp. 43–4.
40 Taylor, *On poisons*, p. 113.
41 Christison, *A treatise*, p. 44.
42 Citing the German chemist Leopold Gmelin, Christison observes that 'it is rare that the suspicious scrutiny of the world now "recognizes in the accounts of the last illness of popes and princes the effects of poison insidiously introduced into the body"'. *A treatise*, 231.
43 Macaulay, *The history of England from the accession of James II*, 5 vols (4th edn, London: Longman, Brown, Green and Longmans, 1849), 1, p. 440.
44 In his course on medical jurisprudence at the 1836–37 University of London medical session, for example, Anthony Todd Thompson indulges without hesitation in retelling poison lore. 'Lectures on medical jurisprudence, at the University of London', *Lancet* 2 (1836–37), pp. 321–2.
45 See chapter 1, p. 33.
46 'The suppression of the crime of secret poisoning', *London medical gazette* 4 (n.s.) (1847), pp. 284–8, p. 284.
47 *Ibid.*, 'On the increase of the crime of secret poisoning', pp. 191–94, p. 191.
48 *Ibid.*, 'On the increase of secret poisoning in this country', pp. 105–8, p. 107. Emphasis original.
49 Alexander Dumas, *The Count of Monte Cristo*, trans. Robin Buss (London: Penguin Books, 2003, orig. 1844–45), ch. 52, 'Toxicology', p. 591.
50 'On the increase of secret poisoning', *London medical gazette*, p. 106.
51 Edward Bulwer Lytton, *A word to the public. By the author of* 'Lucretia', *etc.* (London: Saunders and Otley, 1847), p. 48.
52 '"A word to the public" – the art of secret poisoning', *London medical gazette*, 4 (n.s.) (1847) pp. 242–8, p. 245.
53 Taylor, *On poisons*, p. 1
54 *Ibid.*, p. 3.
55 *Ibid.*, p. 7.
56 *Ibid.*, p. 8. His predicament is made more striking still in the second edition of *On poisons*, where he concludes his discussion with a rather unconvincing *deus ex machina*: 'A correct definition of poison is impossible, and it is so far satisfactory that those subjects which are the most difficult to be defined, stand in least need of definition'. Taylor, *On poisons*, p. 9.

57 Jacques Derrida, *Dissemination* (London: Athlone, 1981), pp. 95–127.

58 Cited in Currie, 'Poisonous women and the unnatural history of Roman culture', in Maria Wyke (ed.), *Parchments of gender* (Oxford: Oxford University Press, 1998), pp. 147–67, pp. 148–9, p. 154.

59 Sennert *et al.*, *Sixth book*, p. 27.

60 See, in addition to Earles's 'Early theories' and 'Experiments', John Lesch, *Science and medicine in France* (Cambridge MA and London: Harvard University Press, 1984), especially chs 4–7.

61 Taylor, *On poisons* (1859), p. vi.

62 *Ibid.* (1848), p. 8.

63 'Deaths by quacks greater than deaths by acts of violence', *Lancet* 1 (1837–38), pp. 666–8, p. 667.

64 *Ibid.* p. 668.

65 S. W. F. Holloway, 'The regulation of the supply of drugs in Britain before 1868', in Roy Porter and Mikulaus Teich (eds), *Drugs and narcotics in history* (Cambridge: Cambridge University Press, 1995), pp. 77–96, and more broadly on the pharmaceutical society and trade reform, S. W. F. Holloway, *Royal Pharmaceutical Society of Great Britain, 1841–1991: a political and social history* (London: Pharmaceutical Press, 1991).

66 P. W. J. Bartrip, 'A "pennurth of arsenic for rat poison": the Arsenic Act, 1851 and the prevention of secret poisoning', *Medical history* 36 (1992), pp. 53–69. It should be noted, however, that as much as they were united in their campaign against the 'unqualified', the relationship between 'scientific pharmacists' and general practitioners was marked by tensions – general practitioner representatives remained concerned that legislative recognition of pharmaceutical qualifications might legitimize and extend their medical advisory roles, while pharmacists, defending a limited advisory capacity as a legitimate and necessary application of their skills, criticized general practitioners for their drug retailing activities. The terms of the Arsenic Act will be discussed later in the chapter.

67 Cited in Holloway, *Royal Pharmaceutical Society*, p. 221.

68 'Deputation to Lord Granville', *Pharmaceutical journal* 17 (1857–58), pp. 13–16, p. 16.

69 'Legislation against poisoning', *Ibid.* 16 (1856–57), pp. 254–61, p. 258.

70 *Ibid.*

71 'Accidental poisoning', *Ibid.* 8 (1848–49), pp. 260–3, pp. 260–1.

72 'Report from the Select Committee of the House of Lords on the sale of poisons', *British parliamentary papers* 1857, sess. 2 [551], xii, 565, 573.

73 Logie Barrow, 'Why were most medical heretics at their most confident around the 1840s? (The other side of mid-Victorian medicine)', in French and Wear (eds), *British medicine*, pp. 165–85. See also J. F. C. Harrison, 'Early Victorian radicals and the medical fringe', in W. F. Bynum and Roy Porter (eds), *Medical fringe and medical orthodoxy, 1750–1850* (London: Croom Helm, 1987), pp. 198–215, and Ursula Miley and John Pickstone, 'Medical

Poison, detection, and the Victorian imagination

botany around 1850: American medicine in industrial Britain', in Roger Cooter (ed.), *Studies in the history of alternative medicine* (Basingstoke: Macmillan, 1988), pp. 140–54.

74 *Botanical journal and medical reformer*, no. 1 (2 January 1847), p. 2. Emphasis original.

75 *Ibid.*, no. 23 (4 November 1848), 196; no. 14 (5 February 1848), 109. Coffin was infuriated when 'allopaths' insisted that his favoured remedy, *lobelia inflata* was a poison, and responded by listing over 100 poisonous items in the standard pharmacopoeia. It is interesting to note that Taylor and Christison testified at a trial of one of Coffin's local agents that this was indeed a 'strong poison', indicating a willingness to put aside definitional niceties in pursuit of quackery.

76 This print was part of a petition file complied by the Home Office on the 1849 poisoning case of Charlotte Harris. The print was sent in by 'a looker on' who, in urging the Home Secretary to commute Harris's death sentence, asked 'How can you put this woman to death, whilst Doctors themselves are at the very head and front of a system of poisoning ten thousand times more horrible'? PRO: HO 18/274/1.

77 Dr Fosbroke, cited in Phillip Nicholls, *Homeopathy and the medical profession* (London and New York: Croom Helm, 1988), p. 85.

78 See chapter 3 of this book for a further discussion of arsenic. There are 480 grains in an ounce, or fifteen and a half grains in a gram.

79 As the *London medical gazette* observed, given that between one-half and three-quarters of all deaths from poison were caused by arsenic, and that 'there are properties possessed by arsenic to which we need not further allude, that render it peculiarly adapted to the purposes of secret assassination', arsenic was an appropriate target of legislative interference. 'Legislative prohibition of the sale of poison', *London medical gazette* 10 (n.s.) (1849–50), pp. 803–5, p. 803.

80 Christison, *A treatise*, p. 172.

81 'Professor Alfred S. Taylor's report on poisoning, and the dispensing, vending, and keeping of poisons', *Pharmaceutical journal* 24 (1864–85), pp. 172–84, p. 178.

82 James Tunstall, *Observations upon the sale of arsenic and the prevention of secret poisoning* (London: Simpkin, Marshall and Co., 1849), p. 5.

83 'Sale of poisons', *Pharmaceutical journal* 9 (1849–50), pp. 160–3, p. 162. In its comment on a pending bill on indecent publications, which was likened by its proposer to poison legislation, *The Times* observed: 'There is nothing intrinsically wrong in the existence of arsenic or of strychnine. Poison is, as Lord Palmerston said of dirt, matter out of its proper place'. *The Times* (29 June 1857), p. 8.

84 For discussion of arsenic as an everyday substance, see P. W. J. Bartrip, 'How green was my valence? Environmental arsenic poisoning and the Victorian

domestic ideal', *English historical review* 109 (1994), pp. 891–913.

85 'The German poison eaters', *The chemist* 1 (n.s.) (1854), pp. 762–4. This story has been recounted in several modern sources, including John Haller, 'Therapeutic mule: the use of arsenic in the nineteenth-century materia medica', *Pharmacy in history* 17 (1975), pp. 87–100, pp. 92–6, and Richard Altick, *Victorian studies in scarlet* (New York: Norton, 1970), ch. 7.

86 'German poison eaters', *The chemist*, p. 763.

87 Taylor, *On poisons* (1859), p. 92.

88 Robert Christison, 'Account of a late remarkable trial for poisoning with arsenic', *Edinburgh medical journal* 1 (1855–56), pp. 625–32; pp. 707–18; pp. 709–10.

89 James F. W. Johnston, *The chemistry of common life*, 2 vols (Edinburgh and London: Blackwood and Sons, 1855), 2, ch. 23, 'The poisons we select'; 'The narcotics we indulge in', *Blackwood's Edinburgh magazine* 74 (1853), pt 3, pp. 687–95.

90 W. B. Kesteven, 'On arsenic-eating', *Association medical journal* 4 (n.s.) (1856), pp. 757–59, p. 757, quoting from Johnston, p. 208.

91 *Ibid.*, p. 758.

92 *Ibid.*, pp. 809–12, pp. 809, 812.

93 'On the alleged practice of arsenic eating in Styria', *Memoirs of the Literary and Philosophical Society of Manchester* 1 (3rd ser.) (1862), pp. 208–21, p. 221.

94 Craig Maclagan, 'On the arsenic-eaters of Styria', reprinted in *Pharmaceutical journal* 24 (1864–65), pp. 615–19, p. 619.

3

Plain matters of fact: making and representing toxicological knowledge

In 1853 the *Pharmaceutical journal* issued an editorial setting out in trenchant terms a familiar complaint about the treatment of scientific testimony at legal trials: 'In the legal profession', the *Journal* observed, 'the all-inspiring ambition is "a verdict". In the struggle for this prize, truth is distorted, fact is so blended with fiction that it appears under false colours, [and] justice is reduced to a mere hypothesis'. Contrast this with the aims of the chemist – the *Journal*'s exemplary scientific witness: 'He is not called into the witness-box as an advocate or a logician, but as an authority with reference to a plain matter of fact on which his knowledge and experience enable him to throw some light'.[1]

Comments such as these operated on a distinction conventionally drawn between legal and scientific modes of generating proof. In court, plain matters of scientific fact are placed in a context where fiction, false colours and the contingent imperatives of a verdict predominate. There is nothing in this depiction that should surprise us. From the first English manuals on expert witnessing, up to the present day, commentators have devoted considerable attention to strategies through which science might survive its legal ordeal. John Gordon Smith's 1825 *An analysis of medical evidence* – one of the earliest tracts specifically dedicated to this issue – warned the would-be experts of their perilous position when facing the 'dextrous advocate', whose principal aim was to 'trick' and 'deceive'. While the scientist might be master of the realm of things, Smith ruefully pointed out that in giving evidence he had to stray into the advocate's sphere of expertise – that is, into the realm of words: 'As we can have little evidence as to thoughts, opinions, or intelligence, but through words, which are their proper signs and medium of exhibition, a witness can in no other way give testimony'. The expert witness, in this view, is placed in an inescapably inhospitable climate in which he must translate his plain facts into a medium over which he is not in full control, and whose primary characteristic is that it yields to manipulation. Smith's advice is simple, if uninspiring: 'Caution in speaking, as well as in preparing to speak, should be observed by him'.[2]

These concerns, echoed widely by those seeking out a stable position for medico-legal expertise, highlight a seeming incompatibility between legal and scientific modes of generating proof. In submitting to the dynamics of the courtroom, toxicologists saw themselves as entering into a domain marked by interpretive licence, the manipulation of things by words.[3] But the story is more complex than this. By interrogating the practices of toxicology, and especially the way these practices are described in specialist texts, the opposition between chemical fact and legal argument becomes less secure than it might seem at first glance. In generating and representing their evidence of criminal poisoning, toxicologists were themselves engaged in a complex communicative exercise: one that placed a considerable burden on their claims to be testifiers of simple fact. Chemical proof, its own advocates observed, was itself a form of language, and its capacity to convey usable units of meaning derived from a complex and often contested manipulation of the constitutive elements of this language.

The core feature of toxicological meaning, its exemplary 'plain matter of fact', derived from the results of chemical analysis. 'The chemical evidence in charges of poisoning', Christison observed in the first edition of his *Treatise*, 'is generally, and with justice, considered as the most decisive of all the branches of proof'.[4] Taylor agreed. Chemical evidence was that 'deemed most satisfactory to the public mind, and which is earnestly sought for by our law authorities on charges of poisoning. The reason', he continued, 'is that in most cases, it demonstrates at once the means of death'.[5]

This did not mean that Christison and Taylor placed exclusive reliance on chemical analysis. In fact, they explicitly distanced themselves from what they saw as a dangerous tendency among continental authorities to regard chemical analysis as the necessary foundation of a conviction in criminal poisoning cases. Although, as we have seen, both Christison and Taylor viewed clinical and post-mortem evidence as historically suspect, they agreed that with a properly modern sensibility, one immune to the lure of the historical imagination, such evidence should be taken into account.[6] Clinical indications, Christison advised, were significant on several grounds: 'in the first place, they are of great value as generally giving the analyst the first hints of the cause of mischief, and so leading him to search for better evidence. Next, they will often enable him to say that poisoning was possible, probable, or highly probable'. Finally, though they can 'never entitle him to say that poisoning was certain, they will sometimes enable him to say on the contrary, that it was impossible'.[7] Post-mortem signs, which in past eras were relied upon 'with even less reason' than clinical symptoms, could also be of some use. While disavowing outmoded surface indicators (e.g. lividity, early putrefaction), Christison gave licence to internally observable signs like localized inflammation and congestion.[8]

Yet for Christison and for Taylor, clinical and post-mortem evidence were subordinate – supplements rather than valued in their own right. Several factors might account for this preference. As practitioners who emphasized their own laboratory skills in court and in texts, it clearly played to their own strengths, and furthered claims for a space of expertise that might bound the heterodox world of poison and its interpretation. But, looking especially at Taylor's remarks about the foundation for chemical superiority, we can discern a more fundamental reason. Chemical evidence satisfied the toxicologist's audience, Taylor observed, because of its capacity to *demonstrate*.

The form of demonstration, and the value attributed to it by toxicology's wider audience, can be gauged by the comments of two of England's leading nineteenth-century evidentiary theorists. As far as William Best was concerned, it was when 'poison is extracted from the dead body by means of chemical analysis' that science served law in its 'most legitimate, valuable, and wonderful application'. 'Of the various chemical tests', William Wills agreed, 'unquestionably those which, applied to the human body or its contents or excreta, *reproduce the particular poison* which has been employed, are the most satisfactory'.[9] In these comments Best and Wills highlight the extraction and reproduction of poison as the chemist's unique contribution to trials involving a charge of criminal poisoning. The value of this contribution lay in its capacity to neutralize the unique terrors commonly attributed to poisoning – its capacity to violate without apparent trace. By enabling experts to present poison in its tangible, material form, chemical demonstration held out the promise of disrupting the poisoner's insidious designs. Through his reproduction of the equivalent of the bloodied dagger in his tubes and retorts, the toxicologist promised to translate this most ephemeral of crimes into a more conventional form of violence.

Medico-legal commentators were themselves fully aware of the attractions of this form of evidence, and its consequent value to the toxicological witness seeking to convince in a court of law. Chemical reproduction,

Christison observed, by allowing poison to be 'lodge[d] in evidence' at trial, 'must obviously be much more satisfactory to the mind of an unpracticed operator, and still more to the unscientific minds of a criminal court and jury – an object which every medical jurist should keep in view'. Christison's emphasis on the practical theatrics of courtroom demonstration was not lost on witnesses called to testify at poison trials, many of whom brought in items from the laboratory (encrusted test-tubes, metallic film on plates, etc.) for the edification of the judge and jury.[10] These were the chemist's unique contribution to a criminal trial, the material embodiment of his distinguishing 'plain matter of fact'.

It is important to recognize that this legal enthusiasm for the demonstrative potential of chemical proof was itself linked to a broader interest in poisoning cases as a special instance of evidentiary theory. For centuries, poisoning cases had served as a core illustration of a distinct category of 'exceptional' crimes (*crimum exceptum*) requiring special consideration. Sixteenth-century legal writers, drawing on traditions established in Roman and canon law, identified poison as one of a number of inherently secret crimes which could not be resolved by the preferred means of direct (eyewitness or confessional) proof. For poisoning cases (along with other occluded crimes like witchcraft and rape), indirect proof, traditionally seen as inferior and supplementary only, was granted self-sufficient status. This, as Barbara Shapiro argues, was the start of a gradual process through which the relative value of direct and circumstantial evidence became reversed. Initially framed as a strict exception to normal proof, by the eighteenth century circumstantial evidence was becoming detached from the special category of secret crime, and was widely regarded as providing a superior, probabilistic form of proof.[11]

According to Shapiro's account, the integration of probabilistic thinking in English law eventually made secret crimes a redundant category. But while it may be true that interest in certain 'exceptional crimes' (notably witchcraft accusations) did decline, and that, for many, circumstantial proof became accepted as a means of attaining 'moral certainty', it is not the case that eighteenth- and early nineteenth-century legal commentators dispensed with the category altogether. Constructing reliable proof from circumstance, they agreed, was a complex matter – one that was liable to error if not carefully managed.

Because of the difficulties attending circumstantial evidence, English legal writers sought out compelling and real-life examples to illustrate its promise as well as its pitfalls, and for this purpose, nothing served better than the 'exceptionalism' attributed to poisoning. As Alexander Welch has shown, the eighteenth- and early-nineteenth century English legal community continued to regard poison as a special category of crime, due to the peculiar characteristics with which it was commonly associated. Poisoning trials, in Welch's words, were dependent on 'the evidence of things not seen',[12] a conclusion that was itself frequently voiced in contemporary legal practice and theory. Two of the judicial opinions most cited as precedents for acknowledging the increased importance of circumstantial evidence, for instance, were delivered at cases involving the charge of poisoning, and the testimony delivered at these and other poisoning trials was carefully reviewed in the leading general evidentiary treatises of the day.[13]

Poisoning figured more prominently still in new specialist treatises, like those of Best and Wills, dedicated explicitly to explaining and critically assessing the value of circumstantial evidence. 'It is in cases of supposed poisoning', Best observes, 'that the nicest questions arise relative to the proof of a *corpus delicti*'.[14] Wills supports this view by introducing his core discussion of 'The essential characteristics of circumstantial evidence' with the following contrast:

> A witness deposes that he saw A. inflict on B. a wound, of which he instantly died; this is a case of direct evidence. B. dies of poisoning; A. is proved to have had malice and uttered threats against him, and to have clandestinely purchased poison, wrapped in a particular paper, and of the same kind as that which has caused the death; the paper is found in his secret drawer, and the poison gone. The *evidence* of these facts is *direct*; the facts themselves are *indirect* and *circumstantial*, as applicable to the inquiry whether a murder has been committed, and whether it was committed by A.[15]

Wills presents this distinction between evidence of wounds and evidence of poisoning as his sole (and thus paradigmatic) example of what distinguishes proof by circumstance. It is in this context that we can understand the enthusiastic embrace of chemical demonstration by Wills and his contemporaries. Toxicological 'materialism' offered refuge from lingering concerns about the shortcomings of circumstantial evidence. Through chemical demonstration, poisoning trials could more closely approximate less-problematic cases of palpable physical violence.

The *absence* of chemical demonstration in an alleged case of poisoning, moreover, could equally serve legal commentators as an opportunity for further reflection on circumstantial evidence. Samuel March Phillipps, a leading authority on the early nineteenth-century law of evidence, used his 1815 *Theory of presumptive proof* to analyse instances of what he regarded as false convictions founded on ill-judged circumstance, or in his terms, 'presumption'.[16] Presumptions, Phillipps explained, were 'consequences drawn from a fact that is known to serve for the discovery of the truth of a fact that is uncertain, and which one seeks to prove'.[17] The law relied on presumptions in matters that afforded no direct proof. Presumptions were thus tools of legal art – accepted pathways for reaching agreement about something unknown. These pathways were grounded in principles of experience, reason, and justice, the most fundamental of which, in Phillipps's view, was that a presumption must be based on a fact already established as real. 'In law', he insists, 'arguments should be drawn from one reality to another, and not from reality to figure, or from figure to reality'.[18]

Phillipps, characteristically, chose poison as his prime example of the misuse of presumptive evidence, a case in which, because of the absence of palpable chemical demonstration, arguments followed from figure rather than reality. This was one of the best-known (and most contentious) poisoning cases of the late eighteenth century: the 1781 trial of Captain John Donnellan for the murder of his brother-in-law, Sir Theodosius Boughton. Boughton, the twenty-year-old first-born of a wealthy Warwickshire family who on his next birthday was to come into a substantial yearly income, died in July 1780 after taking 'the most gentle and innocent' medicinal draught prescribed for a venereal condition. Donnellan's wife was next in line to the Boughton fortune, and Donnellan's actions following his brother-in-law's death – most notably his precipitous rinsing of the medicinal phial – led several to suspect him of having introduced poison into Boughton's draught. Further investigation by the family and its medical advisers intensified suspicion, and Donnellan was eventually brought to trial before the assize court of Sir Francis Buller in March 1781.

In his opening charge to the jury, a statement which itself became a classic formulation of the doctrine of circumstantial evidence, Buller made it clear that he considered this an exemplary case of secret crime: 'You are not to expect visible proofs in a work of darkness', Buller advised. 'You are to collect the truth from circumstances, and little collateral facts, which taken singly afford no proof, yet put together, so tally with, and confirm each other, that they are as strong and convincing evidence, as facts that appear in the broad face of day'.[19] The key source for these 'little facts' was the deceased's mother, Lady Anna Maria Boughton. It was she who administered the suspected draught to her son, and because any

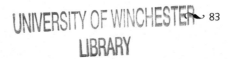

remaining traces of the substance were washed away immediately after use, her ability to identify its distinguishing characteristics took on a critical evidentiary significance. Her sense of smell, in particular, was closely scrutinized. From the witness stand, Lady Boughton stated that at the time she administered the draught to her son she thought it smelled 'very strongly like bitter almonds'. She was then asked to smell a bottle containing the mixture that Boughton's apothecary had intended for his patient, and to declare 'whether that smells at all like the medicine Sir Theodosius took'. When she replied in the negative, she was presented with a phial containing the same mixture into which laurel water had been added. 'This', Lady Boughton declared, 'smells very like the smell of the medicine which I gave him'.[20] In the prosecution's view, this was proof that Donnellan had adulterated Boughton's medicine with a deadly poison, and was guilty of his murder. The jury apparently agreed. Donnellan was convicted of the crime, and promptly executed.[21]

This assemblage of indicators adduced by the prosecution, in Phillipps's critical analysis, represented both in its form and its source all that was dangerous about proofs derived from ungrounded circumstance. Lady Boughton's testimony that the smell of the phial as she remembered it was similar to a substance whose smell was in turn known to be like that of the poison imputed to Donnellan, in Phillipps's view, rested on layers of mediation which could not be accepted as grounds for proof. Lady Boughton had had no prior knowledge of the smell of laurel water, and had only identified it on the basis of its purported resemblance to bitter almonds, a smell she did claim to know: 'One circumstance was supposed from another, equally suppositious', Phillipps maintained, 'and from two fictions united a third was produced'.[22] The Donnellan prosecution, arguing not 'from one reality to another', but from 'inference [to] inference', thus represented a contravention of fundamental evidentiary principle, and the dangers of building a case from shaky circumstance. 'A simile', Phillipps pointedly concluded, 'is no argument'.[23]

In one sense, Phillipps's tract merely serves to underscore, by negative example, the value of tangible chemical proof.[24] Without it, poisoning trials were forced to search for unknown truths by indirect legal methods that were liable, through lapses in logic and lapses in perception, to confuse 'figures' or 'similes' for the 'real'. Presumptions, therefore, were legal tools that required close monitoring, that were open to dispute, and that gained credibility by being tested within the conventionalized arena of the courtroom.

But we can put Phillipps's analysis to a further use, for it suggests a way of exploring some underlying affinities between legal and chemical methods of adducing proof. On the surface, concerns about fictitious inference and misleading similes seem far removed from the chemist's evidentiary offering of plain fact. Yet, on closer examination of the way that chemists and toxicologists operated in their laboratories, important overlaps become apparent – overlaps which set the complaint about legal manipulation of chemical fact in a less-categorical light. The assumption (or, perhaps, rhetorical claim) on the part of experts is that it is only when presenting evidence at trial that they had to contend with the fictions of the courtroom – fictions grounded in the advocate's mastery of the vicis-situdes of language. That is, in the laboratory, the expert works directly with the objects of his scrutiny, unmediated by the play of conventional signs. Yet this is an oversimplification. By the time our toxicological wit-ness appeared in court, he had already gone through an intricate set of representational procedures through which his 'plain facts' were pro-duced. At the core of these operations lay a familiar and self-consciously expressed activity: the 'manipulation' of conventionally agreed signs for anterior realities, the mastery of a language of chemistry.[25]

Examples of this comparison between chemistry and language can be found scattered throughout specialist texts and in popular representa-tions of toxicology, but in my readings none is more striking than that developed by the internationally celebrated German chemist, Justus Liebig. In 1844 Liebig delivered a set of lectures at the University of Giessen, introducing students to the principles of analytical chemistry. Liebig's views were guaranteed a substantial English readership through the auspices of the *Lancet*, which published the complete cycle of lectures, whilst on its editorial pages actively promoting them as exemplary chemical method. Liebig commenced his course with the following reflections:

> All our observations, taken collectively, form a language. Every property, every alteration which we perceive in bodies, is a word in that language . . . The verbal meaning conveyed by the properties of bodies, – to pursue the illustration, – changes according to the mode in which these elements are arranged. As in all other languages, we have in that language whereby mate-rial bodies hold converse with us, articles, substantives, and verbs, with their variations of cases, declensions, and conjugations. We have also many syn-onyms. The same quantities of the same elements produce a poison, a remedy, or an aliment, a volatile or a fixed body, according to their manner of arrangement.[26]

The importance of Liebig's formulation for us is both as an index of the self-conscious linguistic sensibilities at work in the practice of chemical analysis, and as a way of entering into the workings of this language. Understanding this chemical language is predicated on a proper observation of physical change between its elemental units – changes which can reliably signify only to one knowledgeable about its grammatical rules. A full appreciation of differences between ostensibly similar units of meaning, moreover, is of critical importance, an observation that Liebig illustrates through the familiar toxicologically based slippages between the synonymous phenomena of poison, medicine, and disease.

Liebig thus suggests a way of critically reconsidering the evidence offered by the toxicological witness. Instead of seeing him as entering into the perilous use of language for the first time when testifying in court, we might reframe his intervention as an attempt to translate between different, rule-bound, and highly stylized modes of signification. Accordingly, the discussion now turns from tools used in law to establish hidden facts, to strategies adopted by chemists and toxicologists in the first few decades of the nineteenth century to do a similar thing – that is, to gain access to things unseen, and to present their findings not as figure but as real.

To develop this point, let us consider the poison hunter's approach to his key target of analysis – arsenic. Arsenic was by far the single most important poisonous substance discussed in toxicological texts, Christison, for example, devoting nearly 100 pages to it in the first edition of his *Treatise*. 'Of all the varieties of death by poison, none is so important to the medical jurist as poisoning with Arsenic', Christison observed, noting that its ready availability and ease of secret administration made it 'the poison most frequently chosen for the purpose of committing murder'.[27] As a medico-legal object, the term 'arsenic' referred not to the non-toxic metal in its raw state, but to one of its many compounds, arsenious acid, or 'white arsenic'. This substance was formed (most commonly as a by-product of smelting operations) when heated metallic arsenic combined with oxygen to form a sublimate, which was then condensed and purified. The resulting white arsenic – sold either as a fine powder or as a solid mass that could be crushed into a crystalline form – was at once volatile, easily soluble, and highly poisonous. Chemists and toxicologists, recognizing the importance of variables like the form (liquid or solid) and medium in which it was administered, debated arsenic's threshold of toxicity, generally setting it at between two and five grains. Christison, for example, while noting that several authors claimed that two grains were sufficient to kill, stated that the minimum dose he had personally encountered was four and a half grains.[28]

By the early nineteenth century, arsenic's prominence as a poison had led to the development of an extensive battery of tests for its detection, each of which relied upon its own sign system for indicating arsenic's presence. For centuries, it had been signalled through taste and smell – indicators that were toxicology's inheritance from a chemical tradition privileging bodily experience as the basis of reliable knowledge. Taste and smell as tests for arsenic still featured in the early nineteenth-century literature. As William Brande explained to a Royal Institution audience in 1827, when correctly heated, arsenic conveys a peculiar 'alliaceous odour', while its taste 'is singularly nauseous; it creates a peculiar astringent sensation about the mouth and fauces, a great flow of saliva, and a painful feeling in the mouth which can never be forgotten by those who have made the experiment'.[29]

Yet the reliability of this incorporated knowledge was by no means universally conceded by Brande's contemporaries. Indeed, in the same year that he insisted on the unmistakable taste of arsenic, this very point became the subject of fierce debate in the pages of the *Edinburgh medical and surgical journal*. For some arsenic had an acrid taste, for others it was distinctly sweetish, while a third view maintained its lack of taste altogether. In the face of this controversy, an exasperated *Times* editorial declared itself 'astounded' that so simple a matter should have become the subject of public dispute.[30] By the next decade, Anthony Todd Thompson, professor of medical jurisprudence at the University of London, was advising his students that 'every test depending on the senses of taste, or of smelling, should be viewed with suspicion, as much of the accuracy of the judgement that they enable us to pronounce, must depend on the condition of the health of the organs of these senses, and on many other circumstances'.[31]

Early nineteenth-century chemists could also seek proof of arsenic in a seemingly more tangible form – a form more akin to what legal theorists like Phillipps would describe as 'real'. This process, known as the 'reduction test', sought to return arsenious acid to its metallic state by deoxygenating (or 'reducing') it through heat. Adapted for toxicological purposes, this test involved heating matter extracted from the deceased's body in a glass tube, and watching for the formation of a metallic residue on the sides of the tube. Commonly described as the toxicologist's 'crucial experiment', reduction enacted a form of dramatic transmutation through which metal emerged out of undifferentiated matter, thereby promising to expose the shadowy deeds of the poisoner to light. Reduction, however, was by no means straightforward. It was, for one thing, not considered a very sensitive test, in part because a portion of any arsenic present could easily be dissipated in the process of heating.[32] In order for it to work without complex modification, moreover, the material to be tested had to be in a solid state, and free from organic matter.[33]

Given these limitations, chemists routinely based their hunt for arsenic on a group of tests that sought not to reproduce it in its metallic form, but to generate agreed-upon signs of its presence. These processes, collectively referred to as the 'liquid tests', operated on the principle that when arsenic came into contact with one of several specified chemical solutions, it would form a precipitate of a characteristic colour or pattern of colours.[34] These results, medico-legal writers stressed, were reliable alternatives to the reproduction of arsenic in kind, Paris and Fonblanque going so far as to insist that they were not only 'capable, under proper management and precaution, of furnishing striking and infallible indications', but were often 'even more satisfactory in their results than the metallic reproduction, on which so much stress has been laid'.[35]

From a chemical point of view, there was nothing peculiar about the methods employed in the liquid tests for arsenic. Indeed, 'reagents', or substances known to react characteristically when placed in contact with another designated substance, were the principal tools by which nineteenth-century chemists gained knowledge of the composition of unknown matter. 'Chemical Tests or Re-agents', in the words of the popular chemical writer Frederick Accum, 'are called those substances, which, when applied to other bodies, the nature, or composition of which are unknown, *quickly* act upon them, and produce such changes as are sufficiently striking to the senses, and from which the quality or constitution of the unknown body may be inferred'.[36] They are, he continues, 'the compass by which the chemist steers', the means by which he can use ostensibly fixed co-ordinates to navigate the chemical unknown.[37]

This model of chemical navigation was founded on experience and consensus, the relationship between reagent and chemical body guaranteed by reference to rules laid down by a community of practitioners. Reagents performed this function through an agreement among chemists that their actions were reliable and legible. Indeed, the recognized tools of chemical analysis were bounded only by the instrumental purposes of its users: 'It may be readily conceived', Accum observes,

> that a vast variety of substances, provided their chemical actions be well established, may serve as Re-agents or tests . . . By long search and experi-

ence, we have, however, learnt to make a choice of some particular bodies only, the effects of which are rapid, and the application of which requires no skill; and to these bodies the name of Re-agents or tests has been given by mutual consent.[38]

The units of meaning of this consensually derived analytical discourse, moreover, addressed themselves principally to visual sense perceptions. Reagents signified by 'occasioning either a precipitate, a sensible cloudiness, a change of colour, and effervescence, or such other obvious alterations of properties, as experience has proved denote the presence, or absence, of certain bodies'.[39]

Reagents, thus described, are the chemist's equivalent of indirect, or circumstantial, evidence, chemistry itself constituting a collective form of communication utilizing agreed-upon tools to reveal an occluded truth. Looked at in this way, the evidence brought into court by the toxicologist was not a simple matter of fact – a pure unit of meaning that was only then subjected to critical scrutiny on the basis of externally generated rules of 'presumption'. It was, instead, the product of an alternative but symmetrical system of evidentiary signs, derived from conventional procedures through which 'presumption' was made to stand for 'fact'. The results of these procedures, in the case of the liquid tests, moreover, came in the form of sense-based indications that, like the smells in the Donnellan trial, were themselves open to the charge of being figures or similes: subjective signs masquerading as real ones. Chemical writers recognized that language was their principal means of representing these indicators across a range of observers, and that this was itself a limited resource. Joseph Adams, writing in the *Edinburgh medical and surgical journal*, acknowledged that there were insufficient words in any language for the minute differences in many things which are obvious and perceptible to the skilful and experienced observer. 'What a variety of different hues come under the denomination of blue, green and brown!', Adams exclaimed. 'In order to make your idea intelligible, you must produce a pattern, or some familiar object of comparison'.[40]

Chemical texts of the period abound in examples of this effort, producing what to our sensibilities seem a bewildering array of comparative distinctions. Descriptions depended on the recognition of highly specific shades of colour – a purple comparable to the 'bloom of an Orleans plum', an orange similar to 'the peel of a sweet orange', or a 'lively' (as distinct from a 'sad') grass green, for example.[41] These were commonly accompanied by an insistence that the effect was inescapable: reference to the 'brilliance' of a given reaction, which 'once seen, is never forgotten', was a common refrain in contemporary chemical works. In the discourse of chemical demonstration, signs were crystal clear, never murky, cloudy or muddy. It was this quality that seemed to guarantee the unmistakability of the tests, their capacity to circumvent subjective difference and appeal to a universal eye.

Yet the brilliance attributed to colour tests, and its capacity to ground visual evidence in an emphatic language of effect, was itself predicated on material conditions that were by no means assured in the context of medico-legal toxicology. When the analyst was operating on samples that were solid, unmixed, and substantial, tests for arsenic were relatively simple. But, as Christison observed in the first edition of his *Treatise*, in nine medico-legal cases out of ten the subject of analysis was the stomach with its contents, and under such conditions analysis risked being 'enveloped in much difficulty and uncertainty'.[42] Amidst the alimentary canal's typical mix of substances, colour tests tended to lose their capacity to signal with their characteristic clarity. Precipitates might, firstly, be physically obscured by coloured organic material; secondly, colours thought to signal the presence of arsenic might be simulated by analogous reactions between reagents and non-arsenical matter in the body.

These problems had been signalled by a number of highly publicized trials in the opening decades of the century, the most significant of which was the case of the Devon apothecary Robert Donnal, who in 1817 was accused of poisoning his mother-in-law with arsenic. Toxicological witnesses for the prosecution testified that, because the quantity of material available for analysis was insufficient to 'attempt the re-production of the metallic arsenic', they had resorted to submitting the stomach contents of the deceased to two of the liquid tests. Through these means they produced coloured precipitates that for them satisfactorily indicated the presence of arsenic. An Exeter physician, Dr Neale, challenged this evidence by pointing to the deceased's final meal – rabbit with onion sauce – as a source of fallacy. Neale informed the court that he had simulated the presumed chemical composition of the deceased's stomach (onions and phosphate of soda which was, he advised the jury, a common constituent of animal fluids), and had then subjected this to the tests used by the prosecution witnesses. The result, he declared, was precipitates 'very much resembling' the colour indicators for arsenic. With this experiment, he had, in a phrase resonant with the linguistic model common to the discourse of toxicological proof in this period, reproduced 'the source of each substance from which the analogy was taken'.[43]

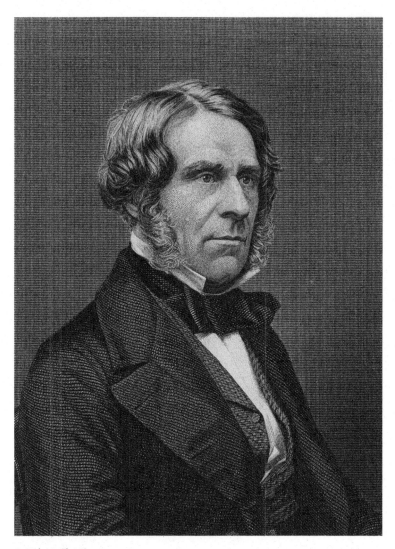

1 Robert Christison

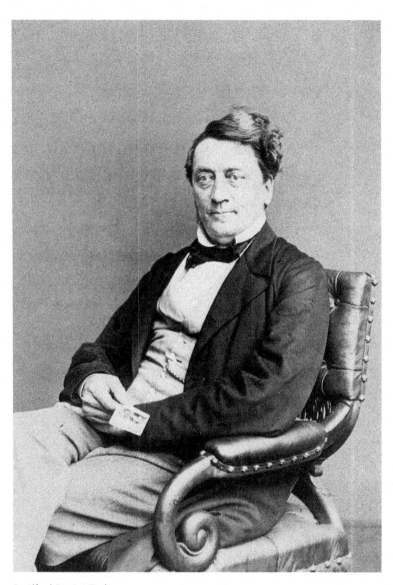

2 Alfred Swaine Taylor

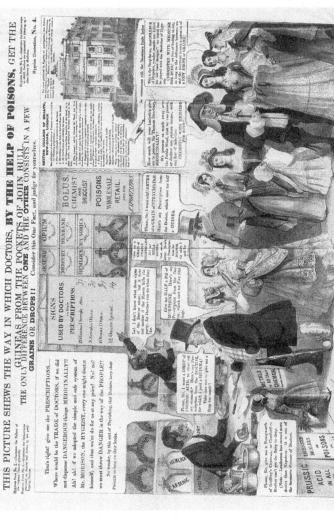

3 Hygeian Illustration no. 4, with historical and fictional poisoners queuing at a Victorian chemist's shop to procure poisonous medicines

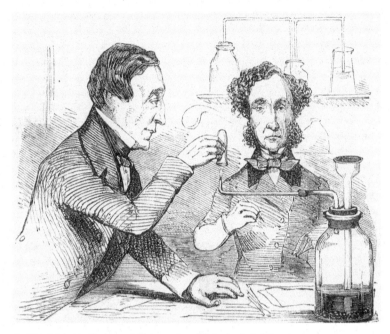

4 Alfred Swaine Taylor and George Owen Rees in their laboratory

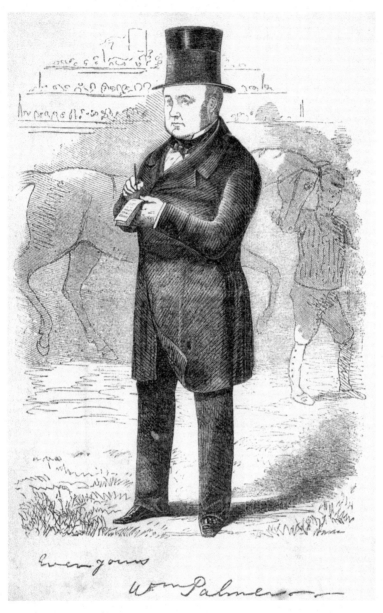

5 Willam Palmer at the races

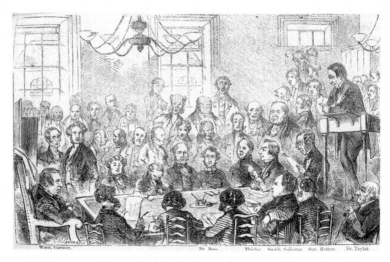

6 Alfred Swaine Taylor giving evidence at the Cook inquest

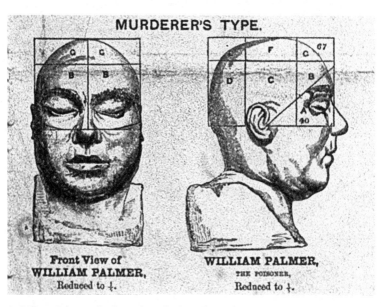

MURDERER'S TYPE.

Front View of
WILLIAM PALMER,
Reduced to ¼.

WILLIAM PALMER,
THE POISONER,
Reduced to ¼.

7 William Palmer's death mask, with phrenological calculations, revealing the prominent trait of secretiveness

The practical instabilities of toxicological signification illustrated by the Donnal case were generalized in experiments conducted by Christison and reported in a lengthy 1824 contribution to the *Edinburgh medical and surgical journal.* 'It is well known', Christison noted, 'that the presence of various mineral vegetable and animal substances in fluids that contain arsenic, alters considerably the action of its liquid tests'.[44] By way of illustrating this observation, Christison subjected the four liquid tests to the trials of the typical British stomach, mixing arsenic with broth, coffee and tea with sugar and cream, port and porter. The results took him far away from the language of stable signification and purity. In some instances, no precipitate was formed where arsenic was present, and conversely precipitate was formed where no arsenic existed. When precipitates formed, they were often 'distorted' in colour, either by the physical interference of the organic medium in which they were suspended, or by chemical reactions between the reagent and the medium which altered its appearance. Under such conditions, language, like the reactions themselves, faded into ambiguity: results were not, as Accum would have had it, 'striking to the senses', but 'very faint', 'pale, dirty', seen through 'a haze'.[45]

To meet this difficulty, several technical solutions were suggested by which a form of simulated purity might be achieved through chemical manipulation. The eminent French toxicologist Matthieu Orfila, for one, proposed the decolourization of animal and vegetable infusions by the introduction of chlorine. Christison, however, argued that such schemes, despite the favourable reception given by many medical jurists, entailed their own dangerous distortions. Orfila's failed on several grounds, most notably because the colour was 'very seldom destroyed so entirely but that the precipitate caused by some of the tests still deviate to a certain degree from their characteristic tints; and although the colour of the fluid be even destroyed entirely, it often re-appears in the precipitates'. On the basis of such distortion, Christison concluded, processes like Orfila's were 'generally useless, often detrimental, nay, sometimes even dangerous'.[46] Medico-legal realities, then, disrupted any claim to a universalist sense perception. However adequate the language of colour might be at a formal level, its utility as a tool of practical communication was limited.

In 1836, the London chemist James Marsh announced a new method for detecting arsenic by 'liberating' it from the material conditions which had hitherto compromised its capacity to clearly signify its presence. Marsh's innovation was based on a familiar set of chemical principles relating to the interaction between zinc, sulphuric acid and arsenic. The combination of zinc and sulphuric acid resulted in hydrogen gas, which in turn exhibited a strong affinity for arsenic, producing the highly poisonous gas known as arseniuretted hydrogen. Arseniuretted hydrogen was a volatile compound that was subject to decomposition under heated conditions. When faced with a compound substance suspected of containing arsenic, Marsh instructed the analyst to mix it with the acid, and then to let the mixture act upon pure zinc. The resulting hydrogen gas should combine with any arsenic that was present, even in minuscule quantities. Having collected the gas in a glass receiver, the analyst would then direct it through a heated tube towards a cold glass or porcelain receiving surface. The hydrogen gas would dissipate, leaving the arsenic to form a deposit, variously described as a crust, film, or 'mirror', on the receiving surface.

Marsh stressed two related – but distinct – features of his proposed process in his initial communication: its capacity, first, to separate small quantities of arsenic from mixed organic substances 'in a pure unequivocal form'; and second, to 'exhibit' the separated arsenic in its 'metallic state, free from the ambiguity' encountered in previous reduction methods.[47] The first statement stressed the principles of chemical attraction, through which the analyst could lift minute quantities of arsenic out of other matter. Separation was not in itself a test, but prepared the ground for the successful application of existing tests by eliminating the fallacies stemming from impurity. The second statement resonates more strongly with the chemical materialism we have been discussing. The process promised a physical outcome – a metallic crust formed on the porcelain receiver – which served as a more sensitive and chemically sophisticated version of the arsenic-hunter's long-standing aim of reproducing arsenic from the body's interior.

Marsh thus presented his process as the solution to the core difficulties that had beset previous efforts to detect arsenic. It is no accident, then, that in announcing the distinguishing features of his process, Marsh invoked the language of purity, the promise of banishing a prior regime of toxicological ambiguity. The production of metallic crusts from minute traces of arsenic mixed in organic matter offered a way of bypassing the murky world of subjective indicators, and of grounding the hunt for arsenic in material fact. We can also understand the enthusiasm with which it was received. With his process hailed as a 'beautiful' intervention by Christison, one 'surpassing the imagination', in Liebig's telling phrase, Marsh was awarded the Society of Art's gold medal, an accolade fully in keeping with his promise to inaugurate a regime of toxicological purity.[48]

The hallmark features of the Marsh process, then, were its unprecedented sensitivity on the one hand, and its demonstrative materiality on the other. This won it praise among leading British toxicologists, and led to its rapid adoption, first in the laboratory, and ultimately in the courtroom.[49] Marsh's most prominent and important advocate, however, was the French toxiologist Matthieu Orfila. Orfila seized on the Marsh test as a crucial instrument for his ongoing efforts to detect ever-smaller amounts of arsenic in mixed organic matter. Its enhanced analytical sensitivity appealed to Orfila, first as an experimentalist seeking to provide demonstrative evidence of the long-debated theory that poison acted by absorption. His success in this endeavour – achieved by using the Marsh apparatus to extract traces of arsenic from the tissues and organs of poisoned human and animal bodies – in turn entailed profound implications for the practising forensic toxicologist. The detection of absorbed arsenic meant that toxicologists could shift their sights from the undigested contents of the stomach to the material folds of the poisoned body. In Orfila's hands, the Marsh apparatus thus represented a signal moment of toxicological modernization. Practically, it lowered the threshold for detection, enabling the toxicologist to detect significantly smaller amounts of poison. Symbolically, physical proof of arsenic poisoning dispensed with the epiphenomenal residue that had been the target of reduction tests. Marsh stains were produced not by the excess of the poison administered, but by that portion of the poison that, by being absorbed, had itself accomplished the murderous deed.

Orfila's investigations thus simultaneously demonstrated the fact of absorption, and constituted it as a new horizon for medico-legal investigation. But the deployment of the Marsh process in the hunt for traces of arsenic carried with it a fresh set of dangers, dangers that stemmed directly from Marsh's trademark sensitivity. Absorbed arsenic, by definition, could only exist, and could thus only be detected, in small quantities. Discovering large deposits of arsenic on the coats of the stomach lead to a reasonable assumption that it had been administered with a distinct, and possibly homicidal, purpose. The detection of fractional amounts, on the other hand, might be explained in a variety of ways. Commercial-grade zinc, sulphuric acid, and even the glass and porcelain materials from which chemistry apparatuses were made, not infrequently contained traces of arsenic.[50] Arsenical medicines, or arsenic absorbed into the body from environmental sources, might also be detected in Marsh's highly sensitive process. The stains produced by trace amounts, moreover, were liable to misinterpretation, not reliably distinguishable from metallic deposits from other sources. Only a few months after Marsh's announcement, the Scottish chemist Lewis Thompson singled out antimony as the metal most liable to be confused with arsenic. Thin films of arsenic and antimony, Thompson observed, were remarkably similar both in their physical qualities, and in the way they might react to the standard colour tests used to confirm their identity.[51] This slippage between arsenical and antimonial traces in the Marsh test was particularly disruptive, from a medico-legal point of view, because antimony was employed as a remedy for complaints such as cholera whose clinical symptoms mirrored those of arsenical poisoning, and as an emetic in cases of suspected poisoning.

The dangers posed by this new regime of sensitive testing were starkly illustrated by a notorious 'error' committed by Marsh's most illustrious follower. Fully alive to the potential fallacies presented by the Marsh process, Orfila initiated an extensive experimental programme designed to investigate and neutralize the potential sources of fallacy. In 1838 and 1839 he published a series of reports on the likely sources of arsenical contamination, indicating how traces formed from extraneous sources might be distinguished from administered arsenic. In one of these reports, Orfila made an astounding announcement: experiments conducted in his Parisian laboratory revealed that arsenical stains could be generated from the bones of bodies that had not been exposed to arsenic in any obvious way. Arsenic, he concluded, might be a natural constituent of the human body.[52]

The implications of this finding were obvious – 'normal arsenic' threatened to contaminate the physical and symbolic purity of the toxicological laboratory. Orfila himself sought to limit the damage, insisting that normal arsenic could be readily distinguished from administered arsenic on the basis of differential properties of solubility. Moreover, in the context of an intense controversy that ensued in Parisian academies and in provincial courtrooms, Orfila rather quickly began to reconsider his faith in the existence of normal arsenic. While never completely disavowing his initial findings, Orfila admitted that he had been unable to reproduce his results, concluding that the subject remained the subject of 'some obscurity'.[53]

British chemical and medical journals, which had closely followed the French debates on normal arsenic in particular, and on the evidence of arsenic poisoning based on 'infinitesimal' results more generally, were less equivocal in their conclusions. A consensus soon emerged that Orfila, despite (or perhaps because of) his experimental virtuosity, had erred by placing too much faith in chemical materialism. He had identified the stains resulting from his experiments as arsenical on the basis of their physical appearance alone, relying on the evidence of metallic crusts that were too slight to be corroborated by more traditional tests. The core lesson drawn by British commentators was that the metallic appearance of the crusts was dangerously seductive. The normal arsenic controversy, in the view of the *British foreign and medical review*, illustrated, 'perhaps as strikingly as any other we can adduce, the dangerous inferences into which an experienced man may be led by relying too strongly on tests applied to minute stains produced from substances'.[54]

In this context, the earliest objection to Marsh – the similarity between slight crusts of arsenic and antimony – was reiterated as a more general principle of evidentiary caution. Henry Hough Watson, a Bolton chemist speaking before a meeting of the Manchester Literary and Philosophical Society in February, 1841, reflected on the lessons posed by the interpretation of thin crusts. Praising Marsh's discovery as a valuable tool for separating mere traces of arsenic from organic materials, thereby 'giving us the power of submitting it to ocular demonstration', Watson insisted that it ought nonetheless be considered as furnishing only 'good collateral evidence'. 'Although a practised eye may discern some difference between the crusts, that from antimony being more silvery and metallic', Watson explained, 'yet the line of demarcation is not easily drawn; for a thin film of antimony looks like arsenic, and a thick crust of arsenic has the metallic appearance of antimony'.[55]

Since Marsh's original announcement, chemists had searched for and published dozens of 'improvements' to enhance its declarative powers, Watson observed, but he remained unconvinced that the fundamental problem had been addressed by any of these 'ingenious' additions. Indeed, Watson cautioned, these additions, while leaving the practical problem largely in place, had introduced new dangers of technical complexity, complications that made the revised tests even less compatible with medico-legal requirements. Watson underscored this point by invoking in unusually stark terms the image of toxicological construction: 'It must, indeed, be lamentable to consider that so much confidence should be placed upon appearances produced by its operation, as to cause a positive conclusion to be arrived at that death was caused by arsenic', he observed, 'when it had been needful to result to intricate manipulation in order to detect the requisite characteristics, and when, at length, only a slight crust or film could be obtained'.[56]

The debates over the evidentiary value of arsenical spots, from our analytical vantage point, can be regarded as a set of contemporary reflections on the breakdown of toxicological signification stemming from a relationship of underdetermination. The relationship orchestrated by the Marsh process between sign and thing was not, under conditions of infinitesimalism, sufficiently secure to guarantee stable meaning. There was, to be sure, nothing unique in this, the problem of underdetermination having featured in discussions of prior tests for arsenic in particular, and of the stability of chemical language more generally. Accum had himself warned that reagents were not altogether faithful to their conventionally allotted chemical partners,[57] while the Guy's analyst George Owen Rees, writing in direct response to Orfila's normal arsenic findings, observed that 'chemistry abounds in instances in which the re-actions of a single test are common to many elements'. This, in Rees's view, placed a considerable but necessary burden on the toxicologist. 'It is not only in relation to our positive knowledge that we must regard this question', he warned.

> We must look to the chances of error from probable causes as yet unknown, and whose fallacious influence can only be avoided, or placed in extreme doubt, by having recourse to the observation of many phenomena produced by the action of several different tests on the substance we are examining – tests which, from their nature, are not subject to the same fallacies as those previously adopted; and whose concurrent testimony is therefore the more valuable.[58]

Rees's resolution of the disruptive effects of underdetermination was thus twofold. On the one hand, echoing Watson's description of thin Marsh stains as 'good collateral evidence', the toxicologist was to have recourse to proof generated not through a single process, but through the corroborative effects of numerous different tests. This was a position endorsed in toxicological texts, and by legal theorists like Best, who declared that 'where several tests, based on principles totally distinct, are applied to different portions of a suspected substance, and give each the characteristic results of a known poison, the chances of error are indefinitely removed, and the proof of the existence of that poison in that substance comes short only of positive demonstration'.[59] Best's endorsement might well be anticipated, since it underscored a form of proof that contemporaries would have readily associated with the courtroom: the corroborative effect of disparate circumstances each of which operated independently from the others. What is critical to note, however, is the way in which this recourse to what Rees himself describes as 'concurrent testimony' threatened to undermine any claim to distinctiveness that might be made of expert testimony in poisoning trials. In other words, rather than being called as special witnesses who had access to a form of evidence that was different in kind to ordinary testimony and that could be superimposed on the trial *sui generis*, toxicologists were now in the position of constructing a proof within a logic strictly analogous to their counterparts in the law. Just as advocates built their cases by assembling a web of testimony that indicated but did not demonstrate the truth of their accounts, so too did toxicologists call on disparate witnesses (reagents) to construct a coherent, but manipulated, discourse of proof.

Rees's second strategy, that of engaging in an ongoing research programme into possible sources of fallacy lurking unknown in the natural world, was also potentially damaging to a vision of expertise as standing above the legal fray, and several commentators were quick to point out this threat. If toxicologists were to follow Rees's stricture to 'look to the chances of error from probable causes as yet unknown', these critics warned, they would be doing nothing less than providing the advocate with ammunition in his professional quest to obscure. A review of Taylor's first edition of his classic *On poisons* captures this sense of peril:

> It seems to be the fashion to ransack the archives of chemistry, and when a substance can be found presenting a reaction common to it with the poison, to set it down as a fallacy, without considering the probability, or, in many cases, the possibility, of its really being in the way. When this is found laid down in a work of medical jurisprudence, it is at once pounced upon by lawyers, who, in profound ignorance of the real value of the so-called objections, bring it forth in cross-examination – sometimes with the effect of puzzling a medical witness ... and sometimes unsettling the minds of an ignorant jury, by a pompous display of sources of fallacy which have no real existence, and thus indirectly encouraging the cold-blooded poisoner.[60]

Taylor's reviewer points to a dilemma faced by toxicological writers in handling the ongoing problem of underdetermined proof. In providing practical information for a readership comprised of potential medico-legal witnesses, texts like Taylor's were responsible for pointing out potential sources of analytical fallacy. Chemical evidence was not straightforward, but was instead the product of a complex and highly self-conscious work of analytical art. Yet in drawing attention to this fact, by, for example, admitting an open-ended search for fallacy as a normal part of the toxicologist's medico-legal responsibilities, or by embracing more generally corroboration as the guarantee of toxicological trustworthiness, expert testimony risked being contaminated by the very contingency that lay at the heart of legal proceedings.

Fully aware of this paradoxical position, writers like Taylor repeatedly inveighed against specious objections raised against toxicological evidence by the reviewer's 'pouncing lawyers', and in so doing sought to stabilize current practice by providing solutions to objections raised in the laboratory or in the courtroom. They were not entirely unsuccessful in this effort. Processes like Marsh's, while never entirely immune from challenge, did serve as functioning pathways for adducing chemical proof. Yet, as the *London medical gazette* observed in the wake of the normal arsenic controversy, toxicologists had to accept a degree of contingency, and the consequences that went with it, as a perennial feature of their activities, one which might vary in amplitude according to time and place, but, barring a chemical closure belonging more to mythic than real time, would be their constant companion:

> The certain test of 1820 is no longer the certain test of 1840; and who can answer what this will be in 1860? Until chemistry becomes a fixed science, and the action of every possible combination of substances has been tried, how can we be sure of our facts, and confidently prove a negative. Every story, says the vulgar proverb, is good, till another is told; and every test is valid, till a fallacy is discovered in it.[61]

Pragmatic though this advice might be, in tying the processes of toxicologist testing so closely to realm of fallacy and story-telling, the *Gazette* simply highlighted the tension underlying toxicologists' appearances in the court of law: their promise of materiality and 'matter of fact-ness' on the one hand, and their need to imaginatively construct a narrative out of signs which were themselves subjective, ephemeral, and open to dispute. Toxicology, rather than bringing stable knowledge to bear upon an otherwise contentious form of inquiry, in this sense simply formed part of the agonistic process of fact-finding.

This chapter has focused on the relationship between legal and chemical standards of proof and evidence. Poison posed special problems for managing evidence in the courtroom – problems that participants looked to chemical materialism to resolve. Yet toxicologists acknowledged limits to their capacity to produce tangible tokens of poison in the courtroom. In developing alternative forms of demonstration, however, their evidence began to lose its claims to distinctiveness. Their 'plain matters of fact', on closer scrutiny, were anything but plain, their force dependent on a complex set of representational practices which implicitly and at times explicitly drew on the language of the courtroom. By tacking between legal and chemical theory, and between the manipulation of words for things and the manipulation of things as words, this chapter has thus sought not merely to shed light on the representational strategies underlying toxicological proof, but to suggest ways of reconceptualizing toxicologists' frustration with their 'mistreatment' in the courtroom. Poisoning trials, which provided medico-legal expertise with a stage on which to display its declarative capabilities, were also events in which the foundations of toxicological proof came under close scrutiny.

The following chapter takes these themes, developed here in a fairly abstract form, and grounds them in the particular circumstances of the most celebrated poisoning trial of the period covered in this book. To conclude the present discussion, however, I want to suggest how the analysis developed above not only allows us to reposition the toxicologist as an expert necessarily interested in the manipulation of signs, but to place this expert in comparative relation to what might be regarded as a competing expert who, like the toxicologist, conducts tests on raw matter in a conventionalized space in order to establish some underlying reality that can be brought forward as evidence. This alternative expert is the trial advocate, his means of testing is cross-examination, his space is the open court, and his analytical object is verbal testimony.

In order to appreciate this comparison, we must return briefly to developments in the conceptualization of evidence in contemporary English felony trials. Legal historians agree that what we now recognize as the adversarial framing of these proceedings emerged over the course of the eighteenth and early nineteenth centuries. What J. M. Beattie describes as the 'old' form of felony trial, elements of which survived into the early nineteenth century, was distinct in several key and interrelated respects. It was short – even a complex case involving a charge of murder would rarely be expected to last more than a few hours. Counsel was typically absent, and there was little in the way of formally introduced testimonial evidence by the parties concerned. It was the judge (and to a much lesser extent the jury) who was responsible for developing testimony, acting as examiner and cross-examiner, and determining when sufficient evidence had been adduced.[62] Moreover, as Stephen Landsman argues, the type of evidence most actively sought was not discursive or dialogic but static, with trials predominantly being 'a search for a determinative piece of documentary proof rather than the examination of evidence in open court'.[63]

This framework had begun to erode by the early to mid-eighteenth century, gradually replaced by an emerging 'adversarial' system. For our limited purposes, two related features of this new procedure are note-worthy: the emphasis on carefully scrutinized oral testimony as the evidentiary focal point of trials; and the pivotal role played by advocates in developing, presenting, and examining such evidence before a more passive judge and jury according to increasingly strict rules of admissibility. Here, the critical interrogation by advocates of evidence provided by physically present witnesses took centre stage. Cross-examination was, in the nineteenth-century evidentiary theorist Thomas Starkie's telling phrase, 'one of the principal tests which the law has devised for the ascertainment of truth'.[64] This observation had, by the time of Starkie's writing, become a core tenet in English criminal law: 'cross-examination of witnesses by *skilled counsel*', Landsman asserts, 'was of such importance that the process was rendered suspect without it'.[65]

The interactive, adversarial encounter between advocate and live witness performed within a rule-bound courtroom space, then, was the modern way to test for legal truth. But if counsel was skilled in the performance of a crucial test, how did this test operate, and in what did this special skill inhere? On the one hand, cross-examination tested the coherence and consistency of testimony. In searching out suppressed presumptions of a seamless narrative, it exposed hidden gaps in testimony. But it was not merely manifest speech that was the object of legal interrogation. Witness testimony was a compound entity, composed of several essential elements that could be subjected to analysis. Legal treatises, reflecting the growing importance attached to the skilful examination of such testimony, urged advocates to attend to signs of an underlying truth obscured by the crude matter of narrative intent. Witness credibility, Starkie advised, could be judged according to the manner in which they delivered their testimony (were they overzealous, evasive, and affecting indifference, or prompt and frank?), and in his view it was the 'viva voce examination', by provoking sensible changes in witness demeanour, that best elicited this evidentiary indicator.[66] Jeremy Bentham, the most committed exponent of trials as live, public, and adversarial contests, was in full agreement. Indeed, as far as Bentham was concerned, the indirect signs elicited from cross-examination were one of the few categories of evidence that could be classified as 'real'. 'How instantaneously the points of agreement and disagreement are brought to view!', he enthused. 'How instructive is the *deportment* exhibited on both sides on the occasion of such a conference'![67]

To get at this level of truth existing beneath the surface, the advocate's principal strategy was to subject witnesses to what was commonly described as 'severe' interrogation. Late eighteenth-century attorneys such as William Garrow and Thomas Erskine attained celebrity status on the basis of their ability to subject witnesses to an intense, if carefully calibrated, verbal examination.[68] Skilled advocates succeeded in their testing operations by utilizing the courtroom as an experimental space in which, by regulating key variables – notably the 'temperature' at which their objects of analytical scrutiny were constrained to react – pure forms might be set free. Garrow, Erskine, and their peers were, in this sense, experts, equipped with their own battery of legal reagents, charged with the task of decomposing raw compounds into the elemental units of truth sought in trial.

What's more, and what brings us back to the discomfited scientific witness we met at the very beginning of this chapter, the testimony most in need of this form of exacting legal test, in the view of evidence theorists, was that delivered by the scientific expert. 'Perhaps the testimony which least deserves credit with a jury is that of *skilled witnesses*', John Pitt Taylor warned in his 1848 *Law of evidence,* adding that 'they do not, indeed, wilfully misrepresent what they think, but their judgments become so warped by regarding the subject in one point of view, that, even when conscientiously disposed, they are incapable of expressing a candid opinion'.[69] It was for this reason that Thomas Starkie, after explaining the value of cross-examination as a means of allowing those present in the court to judge the reliability of testimony on the basis of more than words alone, issued this simple warning: 'These observations apply with peculiar force to all questions of skill and science'.[70] Expert advocates, then, properly had their sights trained on their scientific counterparts.

Notes

1 'Chemical truth', *Pharmaceutical journal* 13 (1853–54), pp. 150–1, p. 150.

2 J. G. Smith, *An analysis of medical evidence* (London: Thomas and George Underwood, 1825), p. 42.

3 Recently, and in response to Anglo-American debate over what critics call 'junk science' in court (that is, adversarially motivated scientific opinion entered into evidence despite its lack of specialist credentials) a growing literature within the field of science studies has been examining how an analysis of the contingent foundations of scientific fact-making, and the social, cultural, and literary technologies that support any claim to scientific credibility, might be used to call into question the assumed opposition

between law and science. For a sample of this literature, and guides to further reading, see the special issues of *Social studies of science* 28:5–6 (1998), edited by Sheila Jasanoff and Michael Lynch, and *Science in context* 12:1 (1999), edited by Tal Golan and Snaith Gissis.

4 Robert Christison, *A treatise on poisons* (Edinburgh: Adam Black, 1829).

5 Alfred Swaine Taylor, *On poisons in relation to medical jurisprudence* (London: John Churchill, 1848).

6 Christison explicitly acknowledged the fine balance that needed to be achieved for a modern toxicology. Although observing that he was 'far from desiring to encourage rashness of decision or to revive the loose criterions of poisoning relied on in former times', he insisted that under specific circumstances, and in the case of specific poisons, clinical and post-mortem evidence were of value. Christison, *A treatise*, p. 132.

7 *Ibid.*, p. 42.

8 *Ibid.*, p. 43. Evidence from the bedside and the autopsy table were of special importance where the evidence of the test-tube failed. Several reasons were given for such failure: vomiting, absorption, and bodily decomposition – Christison observed – might prevent analytical detection. Taylor, with his emphasis on preparing witnesses for the practical contingencies they might encounter in court, gave greater prominence to the factors that might inhibit chemical detection, insisting that – contrary to general belief – positive chemical results were not absolutely necessary to secure a conviction. In the case of certain poisons, for example, toxicology had not yet developed adequate tests, and, even where tests existed, the individual circumstances of a case might make detection difficult if not impossible. This point is developed more fully in chapter 4.

9 W. M. Best, *A treatise on the principles of evidence and practice as to proofs in courts of common law; with elementary rules for conducting the examination and cross-examination of witnesses* (London: S. Sweet, 1849), p. 388; W. Wills, *An essay on the principle of circumstantial evidence, by the late William Wills, edited by his son, Alfred Wills*, 4th edn (London: Butterworths, 1862, orig. 1838), p. 232. Emphasis added.

10 Christison, *A treatise*, p. 195. This form of courtroom demonstration was particularly favoured by William Herapath, the Bristol-based toxicologist who featured regularly in poisoning trials in the south-west of England and in Wales from the 1830s through to the 1850s. Taylor also commonly supplemented his evidence with items from the lab.

11 This was itself part of a broader shift, not only in law but in other branches of enquiry (theology and natural philosophy, most importantly), from a focus on direct testimony provided by a recognized authority as the grounds for demonstrative knowledge, to an epistemology grounded in the corroborative logic of things. There is a vast secondary literature on this topic. The fullest overview of the connections between law and other fields of enquiry is

Barbara Shapiro, *Probability and certainty in seventeenth-century England* (Princeton: Princeton University Press, 1983). Her argument for the primacy of law in the construction of the modern concept of 'fact' is developed in Shapiro, *A culture of fact: England, 1550–1720* (Ithaca: Cornell University Press, 2000). For a philosophical treatment, see Ian Hacking, *The emergence of probability* (Cambridge: Cambridge University Press, 1975). The emergence of probabilistic thinking in relation to the history of English experimental science is a primary theme in Simon Schaffer and Steven Shapin's ground-breaking *Leviathan and the air-pump: Hobbes, Boyle and the experimental life* (Princeton: Princeton University Press, 1985).

12 Alexander Welch, *Strong representations: narrative and circumstantial evidence in England* (Baltimore and London: Johns Hopkins University Press, 1992), p. 25. A substantial portion of Welch's important study of the rise of probabilistic narrative across a range of genres is devoted to poison and theories of legal evidence, and has served as a starting point for my efforts to develop a sustained comparative analysis of legal and toxicological discourses of proof.

13 The first case is *R. v. Blandy* (1752), in which Baron Legge instructed the jury that where a 'presumption necessarily arises from circumstances, they are more convincing and satisfactory, than any other kind of evidence, because facts cannot lie'. T. B. Howell (ed.), *Complete collection of State Trials* 18 (London: R. Bagshaw and Longman, 1809–26), p. 1187. The other case is *R. v. Donnellan*, which will be discussed in detail below. In what is often cited as the first English legal treatise to explicitly mention the place of expert testimony – Capel Lofft's *The law of evidence, by Lord Chief Baron Gilbert* (London: A. Strahan and W. Woodfall, 1791) – the section 'Of proof by experts' is principally occupied with the circumstances of one contemporary poisoning trial. Subsequent treatises make more room for poison: Leonard MacNally's *The rules of evidence on pleas of the crown* (Dublin: J. Cooke, 1802), includes a chapter dedicated to 'Evidence of medical men in cases of poison, while Jeremy Bentham's five-volume contemporary critique of existing rules of evidence contains extended discussions of several poisoning cases: J. Bentham, *Rationale of judicial evidence*, 5 vols (London: Hunt and Clarke, 1827).

14 Best, *A treatise*, p. 166.

15 Wills, *An essay*, p. 17. Emphasis original. Although the first edition discussed the connection between circumstantial evidence and poisoning, that provided in the later edition was more fully elaborated, and is that edition that will be cited throughout this chapter.

16 S. M. Phillipps, *The theory of presumptive proof; or, an inquiry into the nature of circumstantial evidence: including an examination of the evidence on the trial of Captain Donnellan* (London: W. Clarke and Sons, 1815).

17 *Ibid.*, p. 17.

18 *Ibid.*, p. 18.

19 *The trial of Capt. John Donnellan, for the murder of Sir Theodosius Edward Alsley Boughton, Bart., at the Assizes held at Warwick, on Friday the 30th day of March, 1781, before The Honourable Sir Francis Buller. . .* (Bristol: Hill and Blagden, 1781), p. 3.

20 J. A. Paris and J. S. M. Fonblanque, *Medical jurisprudence*, 3 vols (London: W. Phillips, 1823). This text includes an extended appendix of extracts from shorthand notes taken at several poisoning trials, including the published notes of J. Gurney in the Donnellan trial.

21 Lady Boughton was of course not the only witness examined about the phial's contents. The court heard from five medically trained witnesses who, since none of the suspected poison survived Donnellan's scrupulous attention to housekeeping, and since no chemical analysis of the contents of Boughton's body was undertaken (the body being too decomposed for successful analysis), testified principally on the basis of clinical and post-mortem observations. The court was particularly interested in whether they could confirm Lady Boughton's sensory evidence, and four of them made strenuous efforts to do just that. The most illustrious of these witnesses was John Hunter, whose lone dissent to the conclusion that Boughton's death was attributable to poison was in subsequent decades the source of dispute in the legal and medico-legal literature as to whether he represented the face of an ill-prepared or a properly 'modest' expertise.

22 Phillipps, *A theory*, p. 36.

23 *Ibid.*, pp. 36, 37.

24 It is worth noting that in the same year that Philipps's tract appeared, the servant-girl Elizabeth Fenning was tried and executed for attempting to poison her employer and his family. Fenning's conviction was deeply controversial, and became a *cause célèbre*, especially amongst radical political commentators who regarded her case as an example of how circumstantial evidence could be abused by a despotic regime. For more on Fenning's case, see V. A. C. Gatrell, *The hanging tree: execution and the English people, 1770–1868* (Oxford: Oxford University Press, 1996), ch. 13.

25 Observing that nine-tenths of chemical facts are derived from 'artificial means', Michael Faraday embraces the image of the chemical lab as a site of what he calls 'manipulation'. Faraday, *Chemical manipulation: being instructions to students in chemistry on the methods of performing experiments of demonstration, or of research, with accuracy and success* (London: John Murray, 1829), pp. ii–iii. For more on chemical manipulation, see David Knight, 'Seeing and believing in chemistry', *Interface 4: video ergo sum* (Hamburg: Hans-Bredow Institut, 1999), pp. 181–93.

26 Justus Liebig, 'Lectures on organic chemistry, delivered during the winter session, 1844, in the University of Giessen', *Lancet* 1 (1844), pp. 3–7, p. 5.

27 Christison, *A treatise*, p. 172.

28 *Ibid.*, pp. 212–13. There are 480 grains in an ounce, or fifteen and a half grains in a gram.

29 W. T. Brande, 'Lectures on chemistry, delivered at the Royal Institution of Great Britain', *Lancet* 2 (1827–28), pp. 65–9, p. 67. Brande, who in 1813 succeeded Humphry Davy as professor of chemistry at the Royal Institution, was a prominent chemical practitioner and author. It should be noted that despite Brande's comments on arsenic's unmistakable taste and smell, he warned medico-legal witnesses in his next lecture never to declare positively on the presence of arsenic 'unless you get the arsenic and exhibit it by the most unequivocal of all tests, its reduction to the metallic state'. *Lancet* 2 (1827–28), pp. 136–9, p. 137.

30 Christison, 'Account of the medical evidence in the case of Mrs Smith', *Edinburgh medical and surgical journal* 27 (1827), pp. 454–61; Dr Mackintosh, 'Reply to Prof Christison's criticism', *Ibid.* 28 (1828), pp. 85–6; 'On the taste of arsenic', *The Times* (19 July 1827), p. 2.

31 A. T. Thompson, 'Lectures on medical jurisprudence, at the University of London', *Lancet* 2 (1836–37), pp. 448–57, p. 452. Comments like these form a part of a broader trend in chemistry towards what Lissa Roberts has described as the decline of an embodied, 'sensuous' chemical epistemology. For this important discussion, see Roberts, 'The death of the sensuous chemist: the "new" chemistry and the transformation of sensuous technology', *Studies in history and philosophy of science* 26:4 (1995), pp. 503–29.

32 'Unless the quantity of metal be considerable', Paris and Fonblanque's medico-legal textbook observed, 'its metallic splendour and appearance are often very ambiguous and questionable.' (Paris and Fonblanque, *Medical jurisprudence* 2, p. 251).

33 Responding to a process proposed by Christison for preparing liquid organic material for reduction, for example, the *Lancet* worried that 'amidst these multifarious neutralizations and testings, and additions of acid after alkali, and alkali after acid, the arsenious acid will be precipitated without [the analyst's] knowledge and lost altogether'. 'Practical commentaries on Dr Christison's processes for detecting poisons', *Lancet* 1 (1830–31), pp. 545–50, p. 548.

34 In the first decades of the nineteenth century, four substances were discussed: ammoniacal sulphate of copper, ammoniacal nitrate of silver, lime water, and sulphuretted hydrogen. By the time of Christison's *Treatise*, lime water had been eliminated as a viable testing agent.

35 Paris and Fonblanque, *Medical jurisprudence* 2, p. 251.

36 Frederick Accum, *A practical treatise on the use and application of chemical tests*, 2nd edn (London: Thomas Boys, 1818), p. 49. Emphasis original.

37 *Ibid.*, p. 50.

38 *Ibid.*, p. 53–4.

39 *Ibid.*, p. 52.

40 Joseph Adams, 'Observations on morbid poisons, chronic and acute', *Edinburgh medical and surgical journal* 3 (1807), pp. 333–46, p. 335.

41 These descriptions are taken from William Guy, 'On the colour tests for strychnia', *Pharmaceutical journal* 2 (1860–61), pp. 558–606, p. 604.

42 Christison, *A treatise*, p. 197.

43 James Kerr, 'On poisoning with arsenic', *London physical and medical journal* 38 (1817), pp. 92–5, p. 93.

44 Robert Christison, 'On the detection of minute quantities of arsenic in mixed fluid', *Edinburgh medical and surgical journal* 22 (1824), pp. 60–83, p. 60.

45 *Ibid.*, p. 63.

46 *Ibid.*, p. 72.

47 James Marsh, 'Account of a method of separating small quantities of arsenic from substances with which it may be mixed', *Edinburgh new philosophical journal* 21 (1836), pp. 229–36, p. 229.

48 Robert Christison, *A treatise on poisons*, 4th edn (Edinburgh: A. and C. Black, 1845), p. 268.

49 Taylor reported experiments with the Marsh apparatus in 1837, and by the early 1840s chemists were using it as a recognized test in arsenic trials. Taylor, 'Two cases of fatal poisoning by arsenious acid', *Guy's Hospital reports* 2 (1837), pp. 68–83, pp. 75–7.

50 In his original communication, Marsh himself identified arsenical zinc as a possible fallacy, but provided suggestions for countering this by means of rigorous testing of materials used.

51 Lewis Thompson, *London and Edinburgh philosophical magazine and journal of science* (1837), cited in H. H. Watson, 'On detecting the presence of arsenic', *Memoirs of the Literary and Philosophical Society of Manchester* 6 (1842), pp. 590–615, p. 596.

52 These reports were collectively published as 'Mémoires sur l'empoisonnement', in *Mémoires de l'Académie Royal de Médecine* 8 (1840). The controversy surrounding normal arsenic, and Orfila's broader relationship to the Marsh test, forms part of José Ramón Bertomeu-Sánchez's current research. I am grateful to Dr Sánchez for discussing his work with me.

53 M. Orfila, *Rapport sur les moyens de constater la présence de l'arsenic dans les empoisonnemens par ce toxique* (Paris: Bailliére, 1841), p. 43.

54 'Orfila on the means of detecting arsenic', *British foreign and medical review* 13 (1842), pp. 183–97, p. 196. See also 'M. Orfila on poisoning', *Ibid.* 11 (1841), pp. 37–55.

55 Watson, 'On detecting', pp. 595–6 and p. 597. Watson's remarks were reprinted in full in the 1841–42 volume of the *London medical gazette*.

56 *Ibid.*, pp. 598–9.

57 Accum, *A practical treatise*, p. 54.

58 G. O. Rees, 'On the existence of arsenic as a natural constituent of human bones', *Guy's Hospital reports* 6 (1841), pp. 163–71, pp. 166–7.

59 W. M. Best, *A treatise on presumptions of law and fact: with the theory and rules of presumptive or circumstantial proof in criminal cases* (London: S. Sweet, 1844), p. 280. Wills similarly validated corroborative results: 'The concurrence, moreover, of a plurality of characteristic tests, separately fallacious, but fallacious from different causes, may, in connection with strong moral facts, yield a result of so high a degree of probability as to be perfectly convincing, though the poison has not been reproduced'. Wills, *An essay*, p. 233. Taylor's *On poisons* serves as an example of a toxicological treatise having recourse to corroborative testing: Marsh results should be corroborated, Taylor advised, since 'the great object of chemical evidence is not to show a court of law what may be done by the use of *one* test only, by peculiar manipulations on imponderable traces, but to render the proof of the presence of poison in the substance examined most clear and convincing'. Taylor, *On poisons* (1848), p. 348. Emphasis original. For Christison, Marsh furnished 'strong presumptive evidence'. *A treatise* (1845), p. 271.

60 'Mr Taylor on poisons', *Monthly journal of medical science* 8 (1848), pp. 609–14, p. 610. The reviewer cited examples of what he denounced as 'the spawn of this medico-legal refinement', Orfila's 'now extinct normal arsenic in bones' topping his list.

61 'Some difficulties in forensic medicine', *London medical gazette* 1 (1840–41), pp. 410–12, pp. 410–11.

62 J. M. Beattie, *Crime and the courts in England, 1660–1800* (Princeton NJ: Princeton University Press, 1986), ch. 7, especially pp. 340–78. See also two classic studies: John Langbein, 'The criminal trial before the lawyers', *University of Chicago law review* 45:2 (1978), pp. 263–316, and Thomas A. Green, *Verdict according to conscience* (Chicago: Chicago University Press, 1985), and John Langbein's recent *The origins of adversary criminal trial* (Oxford: Oxford University Press, 2003).

63 Stephen Landsman, 'The rise of the contentious spirit: adversary procedure in eighteenth-century England', *Cornell law review* 45 (1990), pp. 497–609, pp. 592–3. While it is true, as Barbara Shapiro points out, that witness testimony played an increasingly important role in jury trials from at least the sixteenth century, this raised numerous thorny questions (concerning, e.g. witness credibility, and the relationship of written to oral evidence) that remained contentious well into the eighteenth century. The search for documentary evidence absorbed most of the attention of the first acknowledged systematizer of English evidentiary law, Geoffrey Gilbert; by the mid-eighteenth century, however, commentators like William Blackstone had begun to emphasize the critical interrogation of evidence provided by witnesses physically present in court. The following paragraphs on the growth of oral testimony and its examination in the first decades of nineteenth century are indebted to Landsman, 'Rise', especially pp. 591–603), and Landsman, 'From Gilbert to Bentham: the reconceptualization of evidence theory', *The*

Wayne law review 36 (1990), pp. 1149–86, especially pp. 1160–86.

64 Thomas Starkie, *Practical treatise on the law of evidence*, 2 vols, 2nd ed. (London: J. and W. T. Clarke, 1833), 1, p. 160. The object of cross examination, Edmund Powell agreed, was 'to sift, detect, and expose'. E. Powell, *The principles and practice of the law of evidence*, 2nd edn (London: John Crockford, 1859), p. 442.

65 Landsman, 'Rise', p. 599. Emphasis original. David Cairns has criticized Landsman and Beattie for overstating the importance of cross-examination in early nineteenth-century trials, arguing that they rely too narrowly on high profile Old Bailey cases, and that they confuse an increasing stridency in examinations with its acceptance as a valid and effective courtroom tactic. Cairns, *Advocacy and the making of the adversarial criminal trial, 1800–1865* (Oxford: Clarendon Press, 1998). Cairns lays greater emphasis on the 1836 Prisoners' Counsel Act, which for the first time allowed defence counsel to deliver opening and closing speeches, in accounting for the rise of modern advocacy.

66 Starkie, *Practical treatise* 1, p. 481. This emphasis on deportment, as Barbara Shapiro's work demonstrates, was by no means new. The seventeenth-century jurist Matthew Hale, for example, valued oral testimony because 'the very Manner of a Witness's delivering his Testimony will give a probable Indication whether he speaks truly or falsely' (Shapiro, *Probability*, pp. 195–7). What does seem new in Starkie and his contemporaries, as Landsman suggests, is the emphasis on skilled cross-examination as an integral feature of trial proceedings.

67 Bentham, *Rationale* 2, p. 470. 'The evidence, and the only evidence, which cannot lie', he suggests, 'is that which, without the intervention of any human testimony, presents itself directly to the senses of the judge. In this case is *real* evidence; and such involuntary evidence as is exhibited by the deportment of a party or an extraneous witness while undergoing the process of interrogation' (*Ibid.* 3, p. 249). Emphasis original.

68 Landsman describes Garrow as the apotheosis of adversarialism, whose methods of cross-examination were at once 'contentious and clever', and 'cruel'. Landsman, 'Rise', p. 564. Contemporary evidence supports such a characterization: indeed, as J. M. Beattie has found, their testing courtroom performances were immortalized in satirical sketches like Rowlandson's 'Being nervous and cross-examined by Mr Garrow'. J. M. Beattie, 'Scales of justice: defence counsel and the English criminal trial in the eighteenth and nineteenth centuries', *Law and history review* 9:2, 1991, pp. 221–67, p. 247. See also Langbein, *The origins*, ch. 5. For a critical assessment of the efficacy of 'contentious' cross-examination, see Cairns, *Advocacy*, ch. 6.

69 J. P. Taylor, *The law of evidence, as administered in England and Ireland* (London: A. Maxwell and Son, 1848), pp. 54–5. Emphasis original.

70 Starkie, *A practical treatise* 1, p. 482. Neither, it should be noted, was this

validation of testing expertise through cross-examination a position held exclusively by law scholars: the medico-legal writers Paris and Fonblanque observed that 'there is a natural propensity in human nature, from which the most honourable minds are not free, to view all questions through the medium of some preconceived opinion; in law and in science it is too often apparent. Hence our law has wisely contrived its modes of *viva voce* examination, in which the judge, the jury, and the counsel, on both sides, are equally empowered to sift the truth, and thus counteract the leaning which any witness may be supposed to have towards the party producing him.' Paris and Fonblanque, *Medical jurisprudence* 1, p. 163.

4

The crime of the age:
the case of William Palmer

We last encountered William Palmer on the scaffold. It is now time to find out how he got there. William Palmer was born in 1824 in the Staffordshire town of Rugeley, the son of a sawyer turned wealthy timber merchant.[1] The rise of the Palmer family from trade to commercial respectability was confirmed by several of its male offspring entering the ranks of the professions – a clergyman, a solicitor, and a doctor. William attended the local grammar school, and on leaving at seventeen was apprenticed, first to a Liverpool chemist, then to a medical man in Great Haywood. In 1844 William was admitted as a pupil at the Staffordshire Infirmary, but soon left to pursue his medical studies in London. After a period at St Bartholomew's hospital in London, he passed the Royal College of Surgeon's membership examination: a standard qualification for those seeking to set up in general practice. With this in hand, William returned to his native Rugeley in 1846, intending to set himself up in provincial practice.

The financial burden of establishing his business would have been eased by the legacy of £7,000 that his father had settled on each of his offspring on his death in 1837, and by the assistance of his mother who had inherited the remainder of her husband's estimated £70,000 fortune. A year later Palmer married the twenty-year-old Anne Thornton, the 'natural' daughter of Colonel Brooke, a prosperous former East India official, and Brooke's housekeeper, Mary Thornton. Colonel Brooke had committed suicide in 1834, leaving property and an annual income of several hundred pounds to his daughter. Another substantial bequest made to Anne's mother was to pass at her death to her daughter. Anne's legacy, however, was arranged as a life-interest only, so that on her own death it would revert to the Brooke family.

Anne Thornton was described in press reports as a respectable, pious, and sober woman, the stain on her character stemming from her illegitimate birth and the suicide of her father seemingly removed by her marriage to the newly established Rugeley surgeon. The Palmers soon commenced the building of an exemplary picture of domestic solidity, producing five children between 1851 and 1854, four of which, however, died in infancy. Palmer himself appeared as a responsible member of the provincial middle classes. He was likened to a hale and hearty 'John Bull' type: stout, ruddy cheeked, and broad and open of face, he also displayed the characteristically English traits of civility and charity, and was often spied with his prayer book in hand. Palmer's embodiment of an earthy Englishness was underscored by the solid, unremarkable features of his home town. In articles designed to demonstrate just how deceptive appearances might be, several journals indulged in ironic celebrations of Rugeley's respectable virtues. One of these imagined a world-weary Parisian who, seeking refuge from the boulevard's 'eternal chatter', arrived at the town's train station. 'Here, if anywhere, he might hope to exhume the simple virtues hitherto buried in the dull dribblings of pastoral rhapsodies. Here he would expect to find a true manly race, softened by the gentle influences of home, and equally free from the brutal impulses of a barbarous and the calculating selfishness of a too refined state of society'.[2] The visitor was soon to be disappointed, anxious to escape from the town's darker underside.

As the imagined Parisian traveller found out with respect to Rugeley's domestic charms, so too, it was discovered, did Palmer's standing as a pillar of middle England belie a more complex reality. His true passion, and increasingly his true vocation, was not medicine but the turf. On his return to Rugeley, Palmer acquired a stable and a string of racehorses, which he bred and bet upon. The initial capital for this investment would have come from what remained of his patrimony, but in an activity so famously draining on capital reserves, and with his penchant for placing losing bets, Palmer quickly needed to search out new sources of funding. Having more or less abandoned his medical practice for the life of the turf, he commenced constructing an elaborate network of financial instruments for raising speculative capital, primarily secured on his mother's and wife's fortunes, and underwritten, as one correspondent sardonically observed, by those '"peculiar people" of modern civilization, [who take] much paper in exchange for a little gold'.[3] Through this increasingly baroque edifice of credit, Palmer was able to expand his stables (which boasted seventeen horses by the time of its dispersal in January 1856) and, despite heavy wagering losses, to appear to honour his local debts and thus to maintain the local face of respectability so crucial for a man of the turf. Palmer, as another paper put it, 'faced the world with a pleasant smile and "kept things going"' even as his finances plunged into crisis.[4]

Here this relatively neutral narrative of events becomes overlain with conclusions stemming from the outcome of Palmer's eventual trial, conclusions reached about how Palmer manipulated his family circumstances in an attempt to keep 'things going'. The first event was the death, in the Palmer home, of Anne's mother in 1849. As a result, the Brooke legacy passed to Anne, but again only for the duration of her own life. Facing the prospect of lost access to this substantial inheritance on the death of his wife, Palmer, in the irony-laden words of the *Leader*, took a remedy 'suggested by certain institutions devised by the commercial spirit of this sensible nation to assuage their grief' – he insured Anne's life with three companies for a total of £13,000.[5] The policies, proposed and in at least one case medically certified by Palmer himself, came into effect in early 1854.[6] In September of that same year, Anne became ill soon after returning home from a visit to Liverpool, and fell under the attentive care of her husband. Her symptoms during her last illness were reported by Palmer himself to William Bamford, an octogenarian local practitioner, as being consistent with cholera, which was at the time rife in Liverpool. She died shortly thereafter, and Bamford duly certified cholera as the cause. Palmer had no difficulty collecting on his wife's policies.

Yet Anne's premiums were insufficient to bear the weight of his accumulated debt. In January 1855, Palmer proposed the life of his elder brother Walter, a bankrupted and notoriously dissipated corn-merchant, to several insurance companies. Despite having been refused by a number of these offices, and despite Walter's long-term and drink-related infirmities, Palmer managed to insure his life for another sum of £13,000. In August of 1855, after months of attendance by his own doctor and his brother, Walter died. At the time of Walter's death, Palmer was reputed to owe £15,000 to his numerous creditors, with a slightly lower further sum falling due within a few months. He therefore immediately dispatched his solicitor to recover the premiums on Walter's life, but this move was blocked by one of the companies, which eventually dispatched the retired Metropolitan police detective Inspector Field to investigate the claim. With a court case pending against him and his mother for the recovery of money advanced on a forged bill of exchange, this delay posed a serious problem.[7]

It is at this point that John Parsons Cook enters the story. Cook was a twenty-eight-year-old former apprentice solicitor who, on inheriting

£12,000 on the death of his father, had turned to the race-track, and had become one of Palmer's long-standing associates, co-owner of several of Palmer's horses and a betting partner at racing fixtures up and down the country. In November 1855 Palmer and Cook travelled together to the Shrewsbury racecourse, where, on the 13th, Cook won a sizeable sum. Cook collected only a portion of his stakes immediately after the race, the remainder of which was payable upon the presentation of his betting book in London the following week. That evening, after celebrating his victory with Palmer and others, Cook suddenly fell ill. He and Palmer returned to Rugeley shortly thereafter, where a restored Cook took up temporary residence at the Talbot Arms Inn, directly opposite Palmer's home. On 16 November, after lunching with Palmer, Cook took to his sick-bed. He died on the night of 20 November, following an erratic pattern of physical distress that appeared to coincide with Palmer's ministrations.

Cook's executor, his stepfather William Stevens, on making enquiries into Cook's death, quickly became suspicious, especially when he learned that Cook's betting book had gone missing. At his insistence, an inquest was called, with a post-mortem examination to be made by local doctors (including Palmer) and a chemical analysis to be carried out at Guy's hospital by Alfred Swaine Taylor. Palmer's reported actions at the post-mortem, notably his apparent attempt to spill the contents of Cook's stomach by jostling the principal investigator as he was opening the stomach, heightened suspicions against him. At the completion of the post-mortem, jars containing Cook's viscera and their remaining fluid contents were forwarded to Taylor for analysis. The contents arrived (despite, as revealed in the subsequent trial, Palmer's attempt to bribe the coach-driver into staging an 'accident' *en route* to London) accompanied by a note from Stevens informing Taylor of his suspicions of foul play.

Taylor, together with his Guy's colleague George Owen Rees, concluded upon analysis that nothing in the appearance of the internal organs would account for death from natural causes. Tests for a wide range of poisons (including strychnine, sought because Stevens had learned that Palmer had recently purchased some from a local apothecary) yielded only a small amount of antimony – a commonly prescribed mineral purgative, but which, if given in repeated doses, could be fatal. In consulting Cook's medical records, however, Taylor and Rees could find nothing to indicate that antimony had been prescribed. Accordingly, Taylor arrived at the Cook inquest – held between 12 and 15 December at the same Talbot Arms in which Cook had expired – prepared to testify only to the possibility of antimony as the cause of death.

In his initial evidence before the coroner and jury, Taylor deposed that, on the basis of the analysis performed, he and Rees had

> no evidence before us to enable us to form a judgment as to the circumstances under which [antimony] was taken by or administered to the deceased, or to enable us to say in this case whether it was or was not the cause of death; therefore, the result is, that we found antimony in the body, which must have been taken while living, but there were no causes of death.[8]

But the testimony of the next witness dramatically altered Taylor's opinion. Elizabeth Mills, the chamber-maid at the Talbot Arms who had attended Cook during his final illness, recounted Cook's reaction to pills given by Palmer on the night prior to and of his death. Mills described Cook's convulsive movements (which included beating his bed with his arms and legs, followed by a general stiffening of the limbs), the wild look about his eyes, and his agonized declarations that he was about to die. At this point Taylor enquired whether any external lacerations were found on the body that may have linked the convulsions to a case of traumatic tetanus. Hearing that no such marks had been found, Taylor announced that he was prepared to give a definite opinion as to the cause of death. Stating that Mills had accurately described the symptoms produced by small doses of strychnine, Taylor declared: 'My belief is that he died from tetanus, and that tetanus was caused by medicine given to him shortly before his death'.[9] The pills, Taylor continued, must have contained strychnine, the only substance in the pharmacopoeia, to his knowledge, capable of producing symptoms like those described. Cook had died in the throes of a tetanic convulsion, and in the absence of any natural cause, Taylor had 'not the slightest hesitation' in identifying strychnine as the only credible alternative explanation.

There was, Taylor admitted, one difficulty that presented itself to this solution: namely, that he had found no strychnine in Cook's body. Yet Taylor insisted that this absence admitted of a scientific explanation. Unlike the more familiar mineral poisons like arsenic, which remained in the body and could in principle be made the subject of unambiguous analytical demonstration, an organic substance like strychnine was liable to be 'so speedily absorbed in the blood that in the course of an hour after the administration no chemical test at present known could detect it'.[10] Despite a sceptical summation by the coroner, during which he recalled to the jury's intelligence that no strychnine had been found, and that

Taylor had come to his conclusions not on the basis of toxicological analysis but on a chamber-maid's description of Cook's dying agonies, the jury returned a verdict 'that the deceased died of poison, wilfully administered to him by William Palmer'.[11] Palmer was committed for trial on a coroner's warrant. One week later, following local speculation fanned by the local and national press, the bodies of Anne and Walter Palmer were exhumed, with inquests following in early January. On 12 and 23 January respectively, the inquest jury delivered a verdict of wilful poisoning, naming William Palmer as the perpetrator. By the end of January, therefore, with speculation raging as to the true number of his victims – as many as seventeen were proposed – William Palmer stood indicted on three counts of poisoning.[12]

Palmer's case gripped the public imagination as no other poison trial had done before. Press coverage was intense from the first reports in December 1855 through to the conclusion of the trial the following June, with editorialists in the lay and the medical press devoting dozens of leading articles to the case. The intensity of national interest was more than matched at the local level. Indeed, so charged was the atmosphere in Staffordshire – 'divided into Palmerites and Anti-Palmerites', in the words of *The Times* – that, in a bid for an impartial jury, Parliament rushed through legislation enabling the trial venue to be moved to the Old Bailey.[13] On the basis of the analysis laid out in the previous chapters, we are in a position to better appreciate the reasons for this unprecedented interest. There were, to be sure, several contingent circumstances that should be taken into account: the unusually long delay between inquest and trial allowed extensive debate about the case to develop; and the resources placed at the disposal of the defence by Palmer's wealthy mother insured that the prosecution would be robustly tested. But these factors would only have had effect if there were something of intrinsic interest in the case itself. William Palmer – doctor, gambler, insurance speculator – amply met this test, his case crystallizing an evolving set of discourses linking poison to the conditions of civilized society, with Palmer himself figuring as the very embodiment of the modern poisoner.

Indeed, the speed and intensity with which Palmer became codified as the archetypal modern poisoner suggests that this was a discourse in search of a referent, with Palmer serving not so much as the originary cause of these concerns than as the perfect channel for their articulation and amplification.[14] Treatment in the daily and weekly press quickly rendered the Rugeley case into a touchstone of poison anxiety, nowhere more so than in the coverage of the weekly *Leader* newspaper. Founded in 1850 by G. H. Lewes and several other like-minded critics as a radical challenge to the complacencies of mid-Victorian prosperity, the *Leader* had for some time been running a featured column entitled 'Our civilization', dedicated to exposing the false securities of English life.[15] The appearances of domestic tranquillity, the writer of 'Our civilization' insisted, were maintained by an increasing array of ostensibly protective measures that merely repressed natural human expression, creating an unhealthy, and potentially malign, hypocrisy.

Not surprisingly, the *Leader*'s attention was drawn to criminal poisoning as an example of this modern disease. 'The Poisoner in the House' appeared on 15 December 1855, not as a response to the events at Rugeley (which had yet to make an impact in the national press), but to two other poisoning trials that had recently reached their conclusions. The article opened with a chilling question for its readers:

> If you feel a deadly sensation within, and grow gradually weaker, how do you know that you are not poisoned? If your hands tingle, do you not fancy that it is arsenic? How can you be sure that it is not? Your household, perhaps, is a 'well-regulated family'; your friends and relations all smile kindly upon you; the meal at each period of the day is punctual and looks correct; but how can you possibly tell that there is not arsenic in the curry? . . . It literally, without exaggeration, is impossible to tell.[16]

Driving poison into the 'well-regulated' hearth inhabited by its readers, the *Leader* accentuated the threat by stressing the sophistication of the modern poisoner, who, though not as courageous his historical counterparts, 'has a greater cunning for concealment'. This new breed of poisoner, moreover, was not a menace generated from outside civilization, but was rather produced from within: 'we enforce order in the streets, and in houses by the strictest rules; perhaps we have in some degree placed restraints upon natural frankness, perhaps our severe regimen tends to constrain the affections, and the true guardian of home, the natural instinct which repels all hatred and envy, sickens and languishes'.[17]

This analytical framework could not have been better suited to absorb and develop the lessons emanating from Rugeley in subsequent weeks. Through weekly commentaries on the Rugeley case, the *Leader* deepened its claim that the institutions intended as safeguards to civilized life provided cover for the modern poisoner. The vaunted mid-Victorian domestic idyll had produced poisoners who, in contrast to the 'brilliant wickedness' of their historical antecedents, 'shelter under the veil of prudish propriety'. This deceptive facade extended beyond the hearth, and into the core institutions underlying mid-Victorian prosperity: 'The very regularity of our lives suggests a means for the malefactor to arrive at his purpose', the *Leader* observed, 'just as the innumerable legal securities for the protection of money transactions furnish opportunities for the forger'.[18] Other 'securities' of modern life came under scrutiny. Science, it suggested, created new problems through its own protective efforts: 'The extension of chymical science enables us to detect the workings of crime with a minuteness and a certainty perfectly unknown to the times of the Borgias or the Brinvilliers; but the same ingenuity teaches evasion of detection and fresh inventions of atrocity'.[19] And what of the watchful professional guarding our health? After detailing the limits of medical securities – the porous boundary between poison and medicine, the ease with which poison could be masked by ostensibly natural disease, the lax standards of vigilance which allowed cases of poisoning to go unnoticed in life and undetected in death, for example – the *Leader* issued this stark warning: 'Give a medical man motives for getting rid of his patient, and it is clear that he has the man at his mercy. Without a metaphor, your medical man can always poison you if he chooses; and unless he is very clumsy . . ., he can poison you without detection'.[20]

For the *Leader*, Palmer provided a singular opportunity to dramatize its critique of mid-Victorian complacency. But, not surprisingly, the issues raised by Palmer's case far exceeded the limits of this analytical perspective. Not only did it resonate strongly with the long-standing themes that marked out the general Victorian discourse on poisoning, in its specific detail the case intersected with a core set of contemporary social and economic debates. The *Leader's* reference to legal securities, money and forgery – that is, to the connection between arrangements designed to regulate economic transactions and their capacity for subversion – are best understood in the context of on-going discussions about the nature of contemporary English capitalism. With the blossoming of joint-stock companies and the gradual lowering of the threshold for investment by reduced share denominations, the commercial landscape of England was undergoing a major transformation at mid-century, in which, broadly speaking, wealth grounded in substantial fixed assets like land was displaced by new forms of liquid wealth dependent on the flow of speculative capital in a largely unregulated market.[21]

On the one hand, these developments represented a liberalization of investment opportunities that, in the context of larger-scale economic reform including the repeal of the Corn Laws and the Navigation Acts, were seen by political economists as a triumph over 'Old Corruption'. However, there was also widespread acknowledgement that commercial liberalization brought in its wake new forms of abuse, a 'ready-money' society in which credit was secured by fraudulent appearances – false company prospectuses, 'puffed' profit reports, the adoption of the trappings of wealth on the part of individuals in search of investors – often supplemented by more direct means of deception such as forgery.[22] The 1840s and the 1850s were marked by waves of fraud scandals, with those stemming from the 'railway mania' of the 1840s being only the most obvious example of a contemporary degeneration of commercial morality. Introducing his account of the infamous Globe Life Assurance Office scandal brought to trial in 1850, the financial journalist David Morier Evans lamented: 'Certainly at no former period of the history of this country has so much importance been attached to show, and so little comparatively, to substance, as at the present time'.[23]

Concern was kept very much alive into the 1850s, not merely by the continued revelations of scandals in the banking, insurance and railway markets, but also by legislative proposals aimed at extending the regime of market liberalism. The most significant of these proposals concerned the establishment of limited liability for investors in public companies. Until the passage of the Limited Liability Acts of 1855 and 1856, Victorian shareholders risked exposure for the full extent of the debt incurred by companies in which they had invested. Seen by political economists as an unnatural brake on the nation's capital resources, proposals for reform had been discussed for decades, and when a government bill was introduced for debate in the summer of 1855, many hailed it as a means of expanding the investing public, enabling small investors to husband their limited resources without fear of ruin. But there was also fierce opposition to the principle of limited liability from those who saw it as a further incentive to fraudulent speculative 'mania'. According to fierce critics in the House of Lords, the bill offered protection not to the solid investor, large or small, but 'to the speculator, who wishes to trade for his own profit but with the capital and at the risk of others'. The main evil, they argued, was its disruption of the balance between the risks and potential rewards of speculation: 'By leaving the hope of gain unrestricted and indefinite a gambling principle will be introduced into commercial transactions, and the risks of trade will assimilate themselves to the chances of the lottery-wheel'.[24]

This invocation of the imagery of gambling in denouncing speculative liberalization was deeply significant. Historians have noted a general, if uneasy, recognition in the mid-Victorian period that new forms of financial and commercial speculation had blurred the boundary between gambling and investment, formerly regarded as polar opposites of the financial risk continuum.[25] Indeed, the crackdown on professionalized gambling embodied in the Gaming Acts of 1845 (which made gambling contracts legally unenforceable), and 1854–55 (which empowered the police to close betting shops and gaming houses), has been viewed as an attempt to shore up the distinction by placing gambling outside the pale of legitimate business activity, an interpretation that was not lost on contemporaries. Responding to the proposed 1854 legislation against betting shops, for example, *The Times* decried the 'puritanical pretence' of the anti-gambling sentiment, claiming that England was in fact 'the most gambling nation in the world'. While free from continental indulgences like roulette wheels and dicing tables, it explained, 'we gamble in the Mart and on the Exchange' – a far more dangerous practice, since it reached deep into the fabric of society: 'the country parson, the schoolmaster, the hard-working, self denying small tradesman, . . . risks the savings of his life and the fortunes of his children on an undertaking of which he knows no more than the next turn of a die, and brings his family to poverty and degradation'.[26] Echoing the contemporaneous critiques of limited liability (and foreshadowing Palmer's use of his family as a speculative resource), *The Times* descried the rippling effects of this chimerical market-place: 'A man assumes the appearance of inexhaustible wealth, buys and buys, and buys again, each time with the credit derived from former but still unsettled transactions'.[27] When the speculation fails, 'father, mother, uncles, aunts, brothers, sisters – all are ruthlessly plundered to save from exposure a "victim" who never had a farthing that he could rightly call his own'.[28]

In the years immediately preceding Palmer's case, then, the nexus of gaming and the speculative manipulation of ostensibly 'prudential' forms of market investment were live issues. Palmer, in this light, served as the perfect embodiment of the blurred boundaries between the two. He was a man of the turf, who bred and bet on proceeds derived from manipulating various sources of credit, largely 'plundered' from his family. But the manipulation which had led him to murder, and to his standing as the quintessential modern poisoner, involved not simple forged bills of exchange, but his exploitation of another controversial form of investment: speculation in the liminal market in human life created by insurance companies.

Life insurance was a booming industry at mid-century, and contemporary reaction to its growth was decidedly mixed.[29] On the one hand, the expanding number of policies could be interpreted as a sign of the onward march of civilized values – of thrift, self-sufficiency, forethought in the provision for one's dependent family, and a co-operative ethos that, for the likes of John Stuart Mill, served as the most 'accurate test of the progress of civilization'.[30] Newspaper and magazine articles sang the praises of the insurance principle. In *The Times*'s view, it was 'one of the greatest blessings of the age', while *Blackwood's* could think of 'no institutions in this country more strictly beneficial to the best interests of society, or more benevolent in their motives'. In these odes to insurance, the male head of the middle-class household was singled out for special attention. Those who took out policies were congratulated for having eschewed indulgence in transitory luxury in order to secure their family's future well-being, while the uninsured were urged to do so as a way of 'removing those harassing cares and torturing anxieties regarding the future, which have so often the effect of embittering existence, and even of paralysing activity'.[31]

But contemporaries also acknowledged an altogether different place occupied by life insurance in modern society. This very same emblematic civilizing office, they warned, could be utilized as yet another form of pernicious speculation, one marked by gambling, and the manipulation of credit and appearance. The origins of life insurance, as Supple and Clark show, lay in a convergence of commerce and gambling, involving both the use of short-term policies to collateralize loans (rather than long-term policies to secure the future welfare of beneficiaries), and the use of policies as a way for gamblers to wager on lives in which they had no direct financial interest.[32] Such practices were ostensibly curbed by the provisions of the Gambling Act (1774), which required policy-holders to demonstrate legitimate interest in any life they proposed for insurance. Yet lax enforcement coupled with a broad definition of 'interest' diminished the act's practical impact, leading mid-century insurance publicists like Robert Vincent to complain that 'prejudice still exists with some that it is a species of gambling'.[33] The use of policies as a means to secure credit, moreover, was a widespread and acknowledged practice, one that company prospectuses listed as an explicit benefit of insurance. A witness to the 1841 Select Committee on Joint Stock Companies questioned the notion that it was the prudent paterfamilias that was driving the burgeoning insurance sector, sardonically observing that 'if only provident people were to insure their lives, half the companies might shut their offices'. Insurance, he continued, 'has become an adjunct to money-lending'.[34]

The implication of insurance in the world of speculation, observers widely acknowledged, was accentuated by the business framework within which the modern system of life insurance operated. Of all the ventures available to Victorian speculators, insurance typified for critics the unwholesome trend towards the manipulation of appearances. Requiring little in the way of tangible capital investment to establish a new insurance office, proprietors were able to trade in the mere semblance of solvency, presenting fronts which masked a hollow reality. 'Nothing is more easy', one cautionary tract declared,

> than for a few artful and needy adventurers – bankrupts in reputation and fortune – to start an establishment of an imposing character in architectural appearance . . Neither is it a difficult task, in these speculative times, to fit up the interior with mahogany-desks and costly furniture, and to place behind them a few clerks, with fashionably-cut coats on their backs, pen in ear, steel-pen in hand, and liveried porter at the door, to give an air of importance, respectability, and pressure of business . . . The British public – intelligent, sharp-sighted, scrutinizing, as it is styled – is mightily deceived by appearances like these.[35]

Newspapers echoed concerns about the 'new' offices springing up at mid-century: 'of all public institutions, a life assurance company is that which may be the longest carried on under false colours', the *Morning herald* insisted in 1852, while in the same year the *Post magazine* lamented that 'the facility with which new assurance offices are set on foot, the tempting promises with which each new scheme is baited ...[have] converted a scheme of infinite utility and philanthropy into one of the greatest speculative projects of the present day'.[36]

From this perspective, insurance represented an especially pernicious form of modern speculation, in that it smuggled potentially ruinous practices into the (middle-class) hearth under the banner of domestic prudence. Moreover, as Palmer's case seemed to make evident, insurance threatened more than mere financial calamity: it provided the institutional framework for the modern poisoner's deadly designs. Under a regime of insurance, the unremarkable lives of ordinary people took on a market value.[37] In comments on the Palmer case, insurance took on an emblematic role, suggesting to many the very essence of difference between 'ancient' and 'modern' poisoning. In past epochs, the *Illustrated times* remarked, poison was the scourge of the court elite. In the modern era, by contrast, 'the crime is a matter of business and arithmetical calculation'. In a commodified world, power no longer resided in rank, fixed wealth, or political influence, but in the manipulation of the market. In the unremarkable lives of the insured, 'the floating capital of criminality has found a new investment'. 'A generous nature may be betrayed into a great crime by passion', it concluded, 'but he who poisons to cheat an insurance office, can have no motive but the pence'.[38]

To be sure, the link between poisoning and insurance was not entirely new. During the 1840s, as we have already seen, burial clubs were widely held up as an inducement for murder by poison. But there are important differences between the treatment of burial-club and life-insurance poisonings, differences that enabled contemporaries to further specify what was new about the threat faced in the 1850s. Burial-club poisonings were considered 'crude' affairs, not only in their means and motives, but also in their institutional context. The proper response to these brutal atrocities was the first and foremost the spread of civilizing domestic virtues. But it also entailed more limited institutional reforms, including the regulation or even outright prohibition of burial clubs themselves. Here, reformers could draw on the counter-image of life insurance as an example of modern, civilized self-help. For decades, proponents of life insurance had been campaigning against the kind of 'ill-disciplined' forms of mutual assistance exemplified by burial clubs and, more generally, by friendly societies. Insurance companies, in this discourse, represented the benefits of professionalism, replacing the local, haphazard, and promiscuous space of the tavern-based club with the abstract space of the urban office, a space regulated not by community sentiment but by rigorous actuarial practices.[39]

Palmer's appearance as an insurance poisoner therefore provided one of many pretexts for reconsidering the relationship between poison and civilization. No longer a laudable refinement on the kind of crude associationism represented by murderous burial clubs, the very refinement represented by life insurance brought its own fatal consequences. Modern poisoning, calculative and sophisticated, had found a natural home in insurance offices trading on false appearances – the semblance of financial solidity, and the promise of sound prudential investment underwritten by a disciplined actuarialism. The paradox was striking, and profoundly disturbing: 'Out of the practice of life insurance – noble fruit of the study of the higher branches of arithmetic', Dickens lamented following the Rugeley revelations,

> which blesses 1000s at their hearths and homes, although the product of an abstract science, – out of an abuse of this element of modern civilisation a new race of poisoners has sprung . . . With life insurance we associate most justly thoughts of all that is good, and wise, and prudent. A more beneficial

result of knowledge is not to be found; and yet it is upon this that nearly the whole practice of secret poisoning now rests.[40]

In this context, Palmer's actions in the overlapping worlds of gambling, insurance, and credit can be seen as an object lesson in the 'shadows' of civilization.

Palmer's subversion of the disciplined professionalism that was supposed to characterize modern life insurance, of course, broaches what contemporaries took to be another defining characteristic of his crimes – his credentials as a member of the medical profession. The 1850s was a crucial decade in the long-running campaign to make medicine a recognized profession, culminating in the passage of the 1858 Medical Registration Act.[41] The act represented a partial victory for medical reformers who in previous years had argued vociferously for a system of medical education and licensing which took into account the fact that modern medicine was, above all else, a science. From this delineation of medicine as a scientific practice flowed a double-edged critique of medicine as it was currently organized. First, critics charged that medicine's status as a progressive body of knowledge and practice was undermined by a retrograde old-guard elite, who used its control of institutional power centres – the Royal colleges and the established teaching hospitals, notably – to perpetuate a system based not on meritocratic attainment of knowledge and skill but on preferment and an arcane notion of medicine as an 'art'. The titular heads of medicine, according to reformers, by holding on to an outdated notion of medicine and thereby refusing to validate the true claim to professional distinction available to ordinary medical practitioners, were in turn encouraging a damaging competition from below – from the 'vile race of quacks' we encountered in chapter 2. By refusing to sanction medicine's scientific standing, the medical elite were giving the public the impression that there was no substantive difference between the knowledge of those licensed to practice, and those who practiced following 'alternative' principles.

The quest for professional validation, in other words, was a quest for public recognition of licensed medical men as a distinct, credible, and trusted group, the disinterested representatives of an acknowledged body of expertise used for the individual and collective good. A system of knowledge-based registration would serve to guarantee the power invested in them, not merely by patients who allowed them to intervene in their bodily well-being, but also by larger entities in both the public and private realms which would look to them to provide vital information – to certify causes of death, or the health of an individual proposed for an insurance policy, for example. Of course, this idealized vision of medicine as a licensed guarantor of personal and social order was itself deeply contested. Controversies surrounding the system of pauper dissection following the 1832 Anatomy Act and the ongoing practice of animal experimentation were only the most prominent examples of a varied and widely held suspicion of medical orthodoxy, a suspicion underscored by medical sectarians like Coffin and Morison, who questioned its monopolistic motives as well as the seemingly benign scientific grounds on which it was based.[42]

Consider, then, the kind of advertisement for modern, scientific medicine that William Palmer made. Here was a licensed medical man – the building block of the very edifice demanded by medical professionalizers – charged with systematically abusing the trusts invested in him. If the suspicions levelled against him were true, he had repeatedly manipulated his medical credentials for malign ends. He had laid the foundations of his crime by acting as medical certifier for an insurance policy that he had himself proposed, and that named him as beneficiary. He had then used his professional position to gain access to his victims as they lay in a vulnerable state, using medicine not to cure, but to kill. His machinations at the autopsy table showed him willing to subvert the solemn medico-legal responsibility entrusted only to members of his profession. His crime, moreover, was effected with all the subtlety befitting a man trained in the science of medicine, eschewing, as the *Pharmaceutical journal* put it, 'the clumsy method of poisoning by large doses of arsenic' in favour of poisoning 'as an exact science'.[43] His science of poisoning, moreover, drew on the latest developments in experimental pharmacology. His chosen agent, strychnine, was itself a notable product of this research field, isolated in a French laboratory in 1818 and put to work by Magendie and others in animal experiments aimed at developing a scientific approach to drug therapy.[44] Palmer the medical man, like Palmer the speculator, thus appeared adept at harnessing all the modern means at his disposal to attain his ends. He was nothing if not a man of his time.

When Alfred Swaine Taylor arrived to give evidence at the Rugeley inquest, he did so representing science's promise to defend civilization against the lethal consequences of its own advances. The initial reviews of Taylor's performance were favourable, so much so that they at times seemed to betray a desperate rush to declare science capable of exposing the secret poisoner's insidious designs. Nowhere is this more evident than in the *Examiner*'s first commentary on the Palmer affair, 'Science in the witness-box'. This lengthy editorial, which was subsequently reprinted in *The Times*, constituted a high-profile assessment of the contest between poisoner and scientist in the wake of the Cook inquest and the subsequent inquest on the exhumed bodies of Anne and Walter Palmer. It was, in one sense, a pure celebration of a triumphalist toxicology. True, the Rugeley inquests had made it clear that 'none of us can be assured against the machinations of the poisoner'; but equally evident and more striking still, in the *Examiner*'s estimation, was the fact that science had made the poisoner's life a 'hell on earth', an infernal wait for the inevitable day of discovery. The scientific evidence on display at the Rugeley inquests, the *Examiner* claimed, had proven that toxicological expertise of late had become equal to the challenge of exposing even the most skilful of poisoners: 'We do not remember any case exemplifying so remarkably the great advance made in our time by science, not only as our helper in every-day life, but as a power bearing witness against crime'.[45]

The most striking characteristic of the *Examiner*'s opinion piece was not so much its professed faith in the efficacy of science, however, as the central and repeated trope of a 'speaking body' that it used to convey this faith. 'The dead woman has spoken, and science has presented itself as interpreter', the *Examiner* proclaimed.

> Not only is the tale of poison told with wonderful precision, but the poison itself is produced in court. The antimony in this bottle, says what remains of the murdered woman, was given to me days before I died; here is the antimony given only a few hours before my death; this again is the poison that ran through my heart.[46]

This passage raises a number of key points. First, it specifies that the *Examiner*'s testifying corpse speaks through analytical demonstration, by bringing poison extracted from the body into court as proof of the crime committed against it. Furthermore, it is not Cook's recalcitrant body that does the speaking, but the more co-operative one of Palmer's wife Anne. A selective toxicological materialism, then, enables bodies to deliver such vivid testimony against their assassins, toxicological analysis providing the opportunity to 'let the dead speak'.

The *Examiner*'s indulgence in corporeal communication serves to highlight the ambiguous powers attributed to modern toxicological demonstration. On the one hand, the *Examiner*'s speaking body provided an opportunity for showcasing toxicological progress. Science at the

Rugeley inquests, in putting an end to the evil-doer's 'old comfort, "dead men tell no tales"', had in some sense confirmed a 'primitive' discourse of proof – the ancient practice of placing the corpse before the suspected murderer, in the belief that it would bleed in the presence of its assailant:

> How vaguely was this foreshadowed in the superstition of our forefathers, whose notion of the best evidence of foul play was to bring a suspected murderer into the presence of the corpse! Precisely the same notion we now carry into effect; but for the supernatural there is put a natural language, which science has acquired the power of interpreting.[47]

The *Examiner* thus insisted that bodies, through the offices of toxicological expertise, could be made to testify not as a matter of superstition but as a matter of science, the invisible and ephemeral weapon insinuated into the civilized social body rendered tangible through chemical analysis. Toxicology, in this reading, had successfully translated the excessive imagination of the past into a usable present.

Yet in another sense, the *Examiner*'s celebratory tableau, replete with speaking corpses and testifying test-tubes, threatened to destabilize the very system of meaning which the editorial sought to uphold, inviting questions about how secure the opposition between scientific and superstitious modes of proof actually was. As the case of Palmer unfolded, the certitudes of scientific translation, the promise of a rematerialization of the poisonous agent, and the declarative voice of the body from the grave, were undoubtedly put to a severe test. Most obviously, the *Examiner*'s model of material demonstration through chemical analysis appeared incompatible with the absence of strychnine in Cook's body. Despite toxicologists' stated insistence that this form of demonstration was not necessary to prove a case of criminal poisoning, commentators were clearly troubled by Taylor's inability to detect a fatal dose of poison. *The Times* struck a typical note of cautious concern: 'What the result of the trial will be no one can foretell. Links in the chain of evidence are wanting – the analysts can detect no trace of strychnine – it may be surmised that the tetanus which ended in death resulted from some other cause than strychnine'.[48] The *Saturday review* was more overtly sceptical: 'How precarious is the evidence, if such it may be called, of learned professors as to the alleged existence of symptoms indicative of a vegetable poison of which it is on all hands admitted that we have no available tests in the present state of chemical knowledge!'[49]

This criticism, however, paled in comparison to the charges made in 'The doctor in the witness-box', an article that appeared in the February

1856 issue of the *Dublin University magazine*. This article featured an extended denunciation of what it saw as the newly inflated ambitions of medical witnesses, who were 'abandoning their position as indifferent auxiliaries of justice and advancing pretensions to direct and administer it'. Far from representing 'a field wherein it is safe to erect a gallows', medical jurisprudence in general, and toxicology in particular, was subject to the vicissitudes of intellectual fashion, popular emotion, and the subjective and metaphysical longings of its practitioners. The 'mysteries of chemistry', it insisted, 'resemble those of religion; faith in them must be entire or void'. Yet the toxicologist enjoyed an advantage over the priest, in that he could 'change at will the language of his oracle':

> Every day new names, sometimes conventional, sometimes expressing a new, often a false theory, are applied to common things, only to be altered upon the day that follows . . . It thus becomes absolutely impossible for the ordinary administrators of the law to test a skilled medical witness, who becomes, in fact, himself, a jury sole, whose verdict is the more fatal, inasmuch as, however he may be led astray by the fantasies of science, the instinct of the chase, or the influence of popular prejudice, he is commonly a man of unquestionable respectability, and often of considerable talents and learning.[50]

In this view, the declarative powers of toxicology represented a new form of faith. Stimulated by fantasy, yet clothed in the garb of modern science, the toxicologist had done little more than add a layer of mystification on to the already formidable mysteries of the modern poisoner.

The anticipated centrality of the chemical evidence at Palmer's trial led others to warn against a different form of mystification, equally dangerous in its effect, although opposite in its cause. This threat did not derive from the undue probative value claimed by science, as the *Dublin magazine* had contended, but from the propensity of its representatives to confuse matters to such an extent that a jury could do nothing other than acquit. The question to be decided in the Palmer case, the *Illustrated times* warned in its issue just prior to the opening of the trial, was ultimately not the value of this or that scientific theory, but the guilt or innocence of Palmer, and the safety of the nation in the face of the poisoning menace. The evidence, it opined, must be made 'plain and popular to twelve average citizens of respectability'. If allowed to degenerate into scientific 'pedantry', truth, justice, and public safety would count among Palmer's victims:

> If poisoning is to be treated of as an exclusive science only, we shall have nobody but here and there a Liebig between us and the grave. We are afraid,

in short, that this trial may be made so much an opportunity for Dr. A. to fight Dr. B. that, between both, the jury may get puzzled and the prisoner off. Not for an instant do we presume to disparage the sacred importance of the scientific evidence, but we can only hope that it will be remembered that it is not *science only*, but the *application of science to a particular question*, which is required.

But, the editorial warned in conclusion, greater than the supposed risk of convicting on less than absolute scientific demonstration was the harm that would inevitably befall English society if the jury acquitted as a consequence of the arcane nature of toxicological proof: 'Fancy a notion going abroad, among our scoundrels, that poisoning is an offence so delightfully refined that nobody can be found guilty of it – so perplexed in its nature, that the chances are you may never be proved to have committed it!'[51]

Medical journals also acknowledged the possibility of tensions between public and scientific standards of proof in the upcoming trial, and devoted a portion of its pre-trial commentary to devising ways to defuse them. The *Lancet*, most notably, urged Taylor and others concerned with the Crown's evidence to adopt a policy of transparency. Requests from Palmer's defence for details of the Crown's toxicological findings should be honoured, and the public should at some level be included in the process of generating the scientific evidence:

Is it not desirable that something of a public character should be given to these investigations? Ought they to be committed absolutely to the private direction of any individual, however high his moral and scientific eminence? Ought they, in fine, to be conducted in secret, with no opportunity for the accused person to check the proceedings, no external observation to inspire the public mind with confidence in the results?[52]

In the midst of such widespread rumination about evidentiary vacuums, scientific pedantry, and the closed world of the laboratory, Taylor himself took the unusual step of issuing a number of public statements in the months leading up to the trial – the most controversial of which came in the form of a reported 'interview' appearing in the *Illustrated times*'s fourteen-page special supplement on the Rugeley poisonings. Henry Mayhew, who had been commissioned by the paper to write an investigative series on the connections between life insurance and crime, published – purportedly with Taylor's blessing – the details of his conversation with the 'learned analyst' upon whose findings 'will probably depend the fate of the prisoner'. Although he subsequently denied

having granted permission for the publication of any information relating to the Palmer investigation, Taylor seems to have taken advantage of
the opportunity afforded by Mayhew to prepare the public mind to properly assess equivocal toxicological results. Taylor, Mayhew wrote,

> requested us to state that although the practice of secret poisoning appeared
> to be on the increase, it should be remembered that by analysis the chemist
> could *almost always* detect the presence of poison in the body, and that
> when analysis failed, as in cases where small doses of strychnia had been
> administered, *physiology and pathology* would invariably suffice to establish
> the cause of death. Of this there could be no doubt, and the fact could not
> be made too public.[53]

In May of 1856, then, toxicology had become a matter of widespread,
and competing, public discussion: opinion in the lay press was divided
between those who warned against alienating common sense by chemical
pedantry, and those descrying the subjective influences at the root of a
detection 'mania'[54]; the medical press seemed to acknowledge the profession's vulnerability to charges of authoritarianism in taking away the
public's capacity for participatory judgment; and its leading spokesman
was to all appearances busily preparing the public to appreciate the limits
as well as the strength of his science. It was in this context that the case of
William Palmer was tried.

Some sixty witnesses – more than half of whom were called to provide
expert evidence in one guise or another – testified during Palmer's
twelve-day trial. Subsequent printed accounts drawn from court
reporters' notes typically exceeded 300 pages, of which well over two-
thirds were devoted to medical and chemical matters, a proportion
roughly conforming to the distribution of coverage in the major press
accounts. Toxicology was by no means the only figure in the drama. The
significance of Palmer's suspicious actions both before and after death,
his complex financial dealings, his efforts at sabotaging the post-mortem
investigations, his purchase of strychnine prior to Cook's death, and
many other considerations, were woven together by the prosecution into
a fine chain of circumstantial inference – one that the defence, of course,
robustly disputed at crucial links. But, as the defence and prosecution
both predicted early in the presentation of their respective cases, science
in general, and the toxicology of strychnine in particular, played the
pivotal role. Indeed, the first day was sufficient for the *Daily telegraph* to
pronounce on the importance to be accorded science in the trial: 'Enough

will be gathered from the Attorney General's speech to show that the temple of justice is to be converted into an arena for a display of learning and skill of rival chemists and physicians'.[55]

These predictions proved correct. From the prosecutorial address which opened the proceedings to the closing words of Lord Chief Justice Campbell's summation, the jury heard a mass of expert testimony, which divided into two main categories: the reasons for the absent strychnine and the significance of this absence for the credibility of the toxicological evidence; and the relationship between the symptoms of natural disease and poisoning, and how this related to the role of clinical evidence in generating proof of poison. Of these two, the failure of Taylor to reproduce poison was the most intensely examined. In his opening remarks, the Crown's lead prosecutor, the Attorney-General Alexander Cockburn, directly confronted this seemingly critical weakness in his case: 'The stomach and intestines were submitted to a careful and searching analysis', Cockburn informed the jury, 'and I am bound to say no trace of strychnine was discovered'. Yet in this case ordinary expectations of what should count as proof would have to be suspended. 'I am told by high authority', Cockburn continued, 'that although the presence of strychnine may be discovered by certain tests, and although the indication of its presence would lead irresistibly to the conclusion of its having been administered, the converse of the proposition does not hold; it is found sometimes, at other times it is not; it depends on circumstances'.[56]

Cockburn proceeded to lay out for the jury the variables that might limit the toxicologist's expected capacity to produce analytical evidence of a tangible kind. The material submitted to Taylor for examination, for one thing, had been significantly compromised: Palmer's interference at the post-mortem table had reduced both the quantity and quality of matter able to be examined; the fact that the initial post-mortem examination conducted by local general practitioners had not been exhaustive also meant that some of Taylor's most vital tests had to be performed on a 'mass of feculent matter' extracted from Cook's exhumed body. These circumstances conspired with the lethal properties of strychnine to make its absence in a body no grounds to exclude it as a murderous agent. The tests for strychnine, Cockburn explained, 'are infinitely more delicate and more difficult of application' than those involving substances typically subjected to toxicology's vaunted powers of re-materialization. Strychnine was 'not like a mineral poison, which may be easily detected and reproduced in specie'.[57] With no such 'crucial experiment' at their disposal, toxicologists were thrown back on the world of subjective phenomena – an intensely bitter taste, black smoky flames, and a series of colour reactions none of which commanded confidence when searching for absorbed strychnine.[58]

Had the strychnine been administered in a large quantity, Cockburn continued, these analytical difficulties would not have posed a significant problem, since rapid death would have resulted from the absorption of a minute trace, and a residue of poison would have remained intact for the analyst to detect. But a physiologically sophisticated poisoner – a licensed medical man, for instance – might introduce the minimum lethal dose, leaving no unabsorbed excess. In light of these obstacles, Cockburn insisted, the absence of strychnine was no proof that Cook had not been poisoned by this agent – a point confirmed by prosecution witnesses. Taylor accounted for its absence first by invoking the inherent difficulties of detecting this poison. He described four experiments that he and Rees conducted between the inquest and the trial, in which they had destroyed rabbits by administering different amounts of strychnine. They detected the poison in only two of the corpses: those given doses large enough to leave unabsorbed traces. He rebutted claims, made by defence experts in advance of the trial, that proper investigation would always lead to detection – charging the experts with placing undue reliance on colour tests. These, he claimed, were liable not only to the interpretive dangers inherent in such tests – especially when conducted on minute amounts of impure material – but also to the difficulties of underdetermination. In his evidence Taylor listed several other substances that would yield 'precisely similar colours as those produced by strychnine'.[59] Responding to a question put by Palmer's barrister, Taylor declared that colour tests were so uncertain and liable to fallacy that 'unless you first get strychnia in a visible and tangible form' – that is, as unabsorbed residue in the body – a properly cautious analyst could not guarantee the detection of even half a grain.[60] Those who claimed the ability to detect strychnine under any circumstances, as Taylor would later insist, were guilty of toxicological enthusiasm.

Debates from the toxicological laboratory spilled over into the clinic, as the symptoms of strychnine poisoning were placed under close scrutiny. Strychnine affected the nerves controlling the voluntary muscles, inducing convulsive symptoms which, Cockburn declared, were 'known to medical men under the term of *tetanus*'. Defence experts, Cockburn warned, would seek to exploit this fact in order to account for Cook's death by recourse to natural causes alone.[61] He insisted, however, that while strychnine symptoms might be clinically described as 'tetanic', there were, for those with the requisite expertise, clear distinctions: 'Happily, Providence, which has placed this fatal agent at the disposition of man, has marked its effects with characteristic symptoms distinguishable from those of all other agents by the eye of science'.[62] In support of this scientifically exploitable providentialism, Cockburn called on leading lights from the metropolitan hospital elite (including the surgeons Sir Benjamin Brodie and Thomas Blizzard Curling, and the physician Robert Todd), who testified that strychnine poisoning could be safely distinguished from tetanus.

Yet tetanus and strychnine, Cockburn acknowledged, did share important features, and in the hands of Palmer – 'a medical man, understanding the use of strychnia and its effects' – this symptomological continuum had been exploited to the fullest extent.[63] Indeed, Cockburn proposed that Palmer had 'prepared' Cook's body for an efficient and masked absorption of strychnine by dosing him in advance with the antimony that *was* found in the body. This, combined with other details of Palmer's medical background – notably the revelation that his student notebook contained a handwritten annotation as to the lethal properties of strychnine – suggested that Palmer's 'scientific' approach had made a substance inherently difficult of detection into a near-perfect agent of modern secret poisoning.

The Palmer defence team, as Cockburn had predicted, focused its attention on Taylor's failed efforts at detection, and on the possibility that Cook had not died from strychnine poisoning, but from natural causes. Taylor's failure, Palmer's lead barrister William Shee maintained, was not due to the peculiar properties of strychnine, or to the manner in which it was presented to Taylor at his laboratory, but to the simpler, common-sense truth that Cook had not been poisoned by it. If Cook's convulsive symptoms had been caused by strychnine, he argued, their suddenness and intensity indicated a pattern of administration favourable to detection: the dose would have been large, the death swift, and the stomach contents undiluted and undisturbed. 'Unless the science of chemical analysis is altogether a failure for detection of the poison of strychnia', he declared, 'never was there a case in which it ought to have been so easy to produce it'.[64] The fact of Taylor's reputed skill as a chemical analyst was thereby turned to the defence's advantage. If strychnine was present, who better to detect it than the renowned author of *On poisons*?

One by one, Shee's expert witnesses, led by William Herapath, professor of chemistry and toxicology at the Bristol Medical School, and Henry Letheby, Professor of Chemistry at the London Hospital and Medical

Officer of Health to the City of London – both familiar figures at poisoning trials in previous decades – testified to the ease with which a skilled analyst could detect strychnine, regardless of dose or its material contamination. Herapath stated his conviction that any dose of strychnine sufficient to kill ought to be detectable by colour tests 'up to the time that the body is decomposed completely'. Letheby, for his part, claimed to be able to detect fractions of a grain of strychnine in the most putrid of liquids, adding more generally of his experience with the detection of strychnine in experimental animals: 'I have never failed'.[65]

In the absence of a clear trace of poison, the question to be answered of Cook's death was whether it could be ascribed to a natural cause. For this, Shee turned from the contested world of the strychnine-hunting laboratory to a consideration of the evidence generated through clinical and post-mortem indicators. Launching an attack on the prosecution's evidence on this front, Shee claimed the Crown's list of witnesses to these questions, culled from the elite of British hospital medicine, were the wrong representatives of science to provide reliable answers. He therefore proposed to tap into another vein of expertise, by calling 'not mere surgeons of hospitals' whose experience with convulsive symptoms was limited to traumatic cases, but rather men who have had the

> opportunity of witnessing and of knowing the symptoms of the class of
> convulsions which constantly attack people in their own residences in the
> dead of the night . . . It is the men who have that sort of experience – the
> general practitioners – men who enjoy the entire confidence of numerous
> families, and have the opportunity of visiting, in the way of their profession,
> the poor at their lowly dwellings, suffering under sudden convulsions when
> affected by serious disease: those are the men that we want to tell us about
> convulsions.[66]

What was required, then, was not a physiology of the extraordinary but of the everyday. When asked, these more humble witnesses duly complied. Although disagreeing as to what Cook's dying symptoms signified, they were as one in declaring that the symptoms could not be explained by any disease process that they had encountered.[67] In his cross-examinations of the prosecution's medical witnesses, moreover, Shee launched a searching attack on their knowledge of the clinical and post-mortem signs of tetanic- and strychnine-based convulsions, repeatedly invoking their own past writings to subvert their claims. Challenging Curling's testimony as to the clear distinction between the gradual onset of tetanic symptoms and the sudden symptoms associated with strychnine, for example, Shee invoked Curling's own 1834 prize-winning essay which had included a report of a clinical case of tetanus involving the rapid onset of symptoms.[68] Interrogating Todd, Shee read an extract from his *Diseases of the brain and nervous system*, which stated that, by administering strychnine to animals, an experimental physiologist was able to produce results which 'exactly imitate the tetanic symptoms in every respect; so that you may at will develop the phenomena of tetanus in an animal by giving him strychnine'. Although protesting that these symptoms, while identical in the experimental context, were not so in a clinical sense, Todd had to concede that the irritation of nerves in tetanus was the same as that found in cases of strychnine poisoning.[69]

In his attempt to uncover the gap between authoritative reputation and actual, legally credible knowledge, however, it was Taylor himself that Shee tested most relentlessly. Acknowledging Taylor as the nation's leading authority on toxicology and the author of the most substantive work on the subject in the English language, Shee pressed him on his actual experience with strychnine in clinical and experimental settings: how many cases of strychnine poisoning in humans had he seen?; how many experiments on animals had he personally conducted? On the first point, Taylor replied that he had never seen a human case of strychnine poisoning (there had been only around fifteen such recorded cases prior to the Palmer trial). Shee sought to equate this admission of inexperience with one of ignorance, prompting the following sardonic exchange:

> Shee: I understand you distinctly to say that as respects the effect of strychnia on the human body you have no knowledge of your own at all?
> Taylor: I have not seen a case; I have some knowledge. –
> Shee: I guard myself; by knowledge of your own I mean personal observation: but you have written a book upon the subject?
> Taylor: Yes.[70]

Shee added to this demystification of the textual 'Taylor' by pressing the flesh-and-blood version on the extent of his experimental knowledge. This was found to be limited both in number (ten, five of which had been conducted over twenty years ago) and in kind (rabbits only, owing to Taylor's fear of dogs). 'Is that the only knowledge of the effects of strychnia poison on animal life which you had when you wrote that book?' Shee demanded. Taylor responded that although his personal experimental base was limited, the existing research literature rendered further testing unnecessary: 'Every toxicologist will not sacrifice 100 rabbits when the facts are all ascertained from other sources; I did not feel myself justified in going on points which I knew were well established'.[71] Yet this eschewal of direct personal investigation, Shee argued, had led Taylor to ignore information derived from animal experimentation that might have provided a vital clue respecting the cause of Cook's death. Autopsies on animals killed with strychnine uniformly revealed an engorged heart chamber, Shee informed the jury, while Cook's heart had been devoid of blood. In opening the case for the defence, Shee sought to contrast Taylor's experimental recalcitrance with the more enthusiastic and demonstrative approach of his own witnesses, who were prepared to present their evidence unmediated by recourse to authority other than the jurors' own senses:

> We will prove to you that the heart of the animal which was killed by strychnia poison is invariably full ... I hope, if you have a doubt about it, that some morning before the Court sits you will desire that a reasonable number of animals shall be brought into one of the yards of this building, and that you will see them die by strychnia, and form an opinion yourselves.

Shee could not have been surprised when Lord Chief Justice Campbell categorically rejected this unorthodox proposal for real-time, transparent toxicological evidence.[72]

Shee's examination of the gap between Taylor's authorial mastery of toxicology and his sparse direct knowledge, it should be noted, intersected with contemporary debates about the protocols for applying scientific expertise to matters of law. Although by mid-century it was a well-settled principle of evidentiary admissibility that, unlike ordinary witnesses, experts could testify on the basis of opinion – and even of opinion not derived from their own first-hand observation[73] – the proper limits of this privilege were still a matter of contestation. In 1851 Robert Christison had sought to settle matters by outlining his views on the theory of expert evidence. There was a pronounced bias in the legal mind favouring testimony based on direct experience, Christison wrote – a bias that betrayed a fundamental misunderstanding of the way that the science of medicine actually worked. Medical knowledge, both in its own domain and as applied to legal matters, was largely built out of the observations of others. Medical 'facts', then, were rare in the legal sense of the term. Medicine instead proceeded on 'opinion': exercises in synthetic reasoning based on mediated observation, the value of which could not be measured by the standards normally applied to legal testimony. Despite the fact that some judges still disallowed knowledge derived from sources other than direct personal observation (particularly knowledge gleaned from published authorities), recourse to textual authority, in

Christison's view, indicated strength in the witness rather than deficiency. A person of true learning, relying on 'the facts and principles derived from the classified testimony of hundreds of prior observers', reasoned more soundly than one who, 'affecting to despise learning, boasts that he relies only upon his own narrow opportunities of direct experience'. Christison illustrated this claim by a case of arsenic poisoning that he had once been called upon to investigate. Although he had not previously seen anyone during life who had taken arsenic, 'by frequent reading, lecturing, and writing on the subject, the varied forms of arsenical poisoning were as familiar to me as if they were all marshalled before my eyes'.[74] In his evidence, Taylor was calling on this very same disciplined toxicological imagination. From a modern medico-legal point of view, there was nothing extraordinary in Taylor's claims, either as author or authority.

Shee's demand that the jury draw the opposite conclusion from his examination of Taylor – namely, that the famed toxicologist 'has not any knowledge as to the effects of strychnia more than any of us' – in this sense challenged the very claims to disembodied and professionally sanctioned authority that medical jurists were seeking to consolidate.[75] In this he sought to do what legal theorists like Starkie and John Pitt Taylor had singled out as the advocate's most important task, that of probing, viva voce, witnesses – especially expert witnesses – to determine the true foundations of their knowledge. What he purported to have found was a prosecution case that traded on the very dangers that legal writers had attributed to scientific witnesses: inflated reputation which masked a conscious or unconscious 'partisanship'.

Again, Taylor was the principal target of Shee's charge. Having over-reached his limited knowledge of strychnine, Taylor had found himself upon a legal stage where he had to defend his personal and professional reputation at the expense of his own science. From the very beginning of his association with the case, Shee maintained, Taylor had been the quintessential partisan. Taylor's initial examination had been biased by the stepfather's suspicions that Cook had not died a natural death. His performance at the Talbot Arms confirmed him as an interested party. Having staked his credentials as an expert witness on a highly speculative theory supported by mere 'taproom gossip', he had publicly backed himself into a corner: 'That opinion was delivered, was irrevocable. [sic] By it Taylor's reputation was staked against Palmer's life'.[76] Shee charged that following the inquest, when concerns were raised about the absence of strychnine, Taylor had transgressed professional norms by opening up his laboratory to the press in a deliberate attempt to manipulate public opinion, inviting Mayhew to report that strychnine was often chemically untraceable. 'Did you not know perfectly well', Shee demanded of Taylor, 'in this month of February, just after the shock which the country had received about these Rugeley murders, or imputations of murder, that your interview on the subject of poison might be taken to apply to what was then full in the public mind?'[77]

Despite the obvious bias of Taylor's evidence, Shee worried aloud, it might well prove effective. This was because, as had been the prosecution's intention, the influence of prestige threatened to obscure the practical deficiencies in its scientific evidence. Deference to institutionalized metropolitan medicine, according to Shee, explained why Taylor's 'audacious' charge at the Talbot Arms had swayed the inquest jury. All present at the inquest, Shee argued, were 'impressed with the idea that whatever the doctor that has come from London, that whatever Dr Alfred Swaine Taylor says, must be true; if he says it is poison, poison it is'.[78] This same deference then ensured that the jury's finding would meet with general approval:

> Instantly followed by the verdict of wilful murder, it flew upon the wings of the press into every house in the United Kingdom. It became known that, according to the opinion of a man whose whole life had been devoted to science, a gentleman of personal character perfectly unimpeached, a man who stood well with his friends in the medical profession . . . that, according to his opinion, Cook's death had been caused by strychnine.[79]

The subsequent public discussion of the case in the build-up to the trial had only fanned the flames. Recalling the imagery of an infallible toxicology that had marked early reports of the Rugeley affair, Shee complained that 'for six long months, under the sanction and upon the authority of science, an opinion has universally prevailed that the voice of the blood of John Parsons Cook was crying up unto us from the ground'.[80]

From his examination of Taylor, Shee had hoped to demonstrate that the greatest threat represented at the trial was not the alleged medical poisoner in the dock, but the irresponsible toxicological detective, whose own investment in the case threatened to tarnish his science. In a much-quoted warning to the jurors, Shee urged them to consider what would happen if Taylor's brand of expertise won the day, 'if science is admitted to dogmatise in our courts – science not exact in its nature – science not successful, but baffled even by its own tests – science bearing upon its forehead the motto that "a little learning is a dangerous thing"'.[81] If, on the basis of his own arcane and suspect standards of proof, and against the norms of common sense, Taylor were allowed to prevail, Palmer would be only the first of those to suffer by the verdict.

The charge of partisan expertise was not confined to the defence case. In his summation Cockburn urged the jury to consider the attempts by Palmer's side to 'confound' the symptoms of strychnine and tetanus, and especially to minimize the difficulties of detecting strychnine, as the claims of 'retained' witnesses. 'No parties can be more thoroughgoing partisans than scientific men who have once taken up a case', he declared, illustrating this general observation with the show of toxicological certainty presented by the likes of Herapath and Letheby: 'after they have been retained for this case, and desire that their experiments should have a certain result, they take good care to have doses large enough to leave a small portion in the stomach'. Invoking the spectre of objectivity betrayed, he professed an abhorrence of 'the traffic in testimony to which I regret to say some men of science sometimes permit themselves to condescend'.[82] The trial of William Palmer, clearly, had done little to promote either the image of toxicology as a stable body of authoritative knowledge, or a harmonious consensus about the conditions under which science testified in courts of law.

William Palmer was convicted on 27 May for the murder of John Parsons Cook, and was executed at Stafford two weeks later. Although, in accordance with legal form, the verdict did not specify the manner in which Palmer was supposed to have dispatched Cook, no one was in any doubt that the prosecution's charge of strychnine poisoning had been the grounds for conviction. Indeed, the jury had been instructed by Lord Chief Justice Campbell to deliberate on this ground alone: 'Do not find a verdict of *guilty* unless you believe that the strychnine was administered to the deceased by the prisoner at the bar'.[83]

As he had done throughout the previous six months, Palmer arrested the attention of the nation as he mounted the scaffold. A crowd estimated at up to 50,000 gathered for the event, hoping to catch a glimpse of the condemned poisoner and to hear his last utterance. Here he delivered the enigmatic statement with which this book opened. Palmer's dying words were emblematic of the long shadow that his trial was to cast over the world of poison detection in the years that followed. It is to the legacy of his extraordinary trial that the final chapter of this book now turns.

Note

1 The following account of Palmer's life is drawn from an array of contemporary sources, including newspaper and journal articles, trial reports, and commemorative accounts such as the massive entry for the 1856 *Annual register*, which ran to more than 200 pages. Palmer's case has also been covered in some detail in modern academic texts, notably Richard Altick's *Victorian studies in scarlet* (New York: Norton, 1970), ch. 7, and Thomas Boyle, *Black swine in the sewers of Hampstead: beneath the surface of Victorian sensationalism* (London: Penguin, 1989), chs 8–9.

2 'The Rugeley poisonings', *Leader* 7 (19 January 1856), pp. 52–5, p. 52.

3 *Ibid.*

4 'The Rugeley tragedies', *Illustrated London news* (26 January 1856), p. 87.

5 'The Rugeley poisonings', *Leader* 7, p. 52.

6 PRO HO 45/6260/6 contains papers sent by the Liverpool and London Fire and Life Insurance Company relating to the £5,000 policy taken out on Anne Palmer, and includes the medical declaration completed and signed by William Palmer as his wife's attendant.

7 The civil case against Palmer and his mother (involved as the purported guarantor of the bill of exchange) is a fascinating one in its own right, the highpoint being Palmer's admission that the bill had been forged, not by him but by his late wife Anne. See the coverage of 'Padwick v. Sarah Palmer' in *The Times* (22 January 1856), p. 8. Field had gained notoriety as the subject of Charles Dickens's studies of London's detective police, especially 'On duty with Inspector Field' (*Household words* 3 (1851), pp. 265–70), and is considered the prototype for Inspector Bucket in *Bleak house*.

8 'Alleged case of poisoning by strychnine', *Lancet* 2 (1855), pp. 617–20, p. 619.

9 *Ibid.*

10 *Ibid.*

11 *Ibid.*, p. 620.

12 Although Palmer was indicted on three counts of poisoning by Rugeley inquest juries, his trial was for Cook's murder only, although the charges in the deaths of Anne and Walter remained outstanding if the Cook charge failed. However, all three inquests often tended to be blurred together in public comment on the 'Rugeley poisoning case'.

13 *The Times* (25 January 1856) p. 7; Central Criminal Court Act of 1856 [19 & 20 Vict. cap. 16].

14 As an example of the case's speed of impact, even before the conclusion of the first of the Rugeley inquests, a short story appeared in *Bentley's miscellany* featuring a medical poisoner who used strychnine to further a plot involving insurance. 'A draught of poison', *Bentley's miscellany* 38 (1855), pp. 266–80.

15 For an account of the *Leader*, see Alan Brick, '*The Leader*: organ of radicalism', Yale University Ph.D. dissertation, 1957; for the *Leader*'s commentaries on Palmer, see Boyle, *Black swine*.

16 'The poisoner in the house', *Leader* 6 (15 December 1855), pp. 1199–200, p. 1199. The two cases under discussion both involved a charge of poison levelled against middle-class men: Joseph Wooler for the murder of his wife by slow poisoning (see ch. 2), and Thomas Tutton for attempting to poison his wealthy father, allegedly to secure his inheritance. Both cases, though ending in acquittals, raised issues which would take on more pressing dimensions with Palmer – for example, Wooler's familiarity with medicines, and Tutton's 'irregular' habits which stimulated his need for 'ready-money'.

17 *Ibid.*, p. 1200.

18 'Poison in the prescription', *Ibid.* 6 (22 December 1855), p. 1224.

19 'A respectable neighbourhood', *Ibid.* 7 (26 January 1856).

20 'Poison in the prescription', *Ibid.*, p. 1224. Others agreed that the spectre of the medical poisoner represented a critical turn in history of poisoning: according to the *Saturday review*, the Wooler and Palmer cases 'both present one novel and startling feature. They attach suspicion to the administration of medicine'. 'Can it be true', it asked, 'that the prescription is used as the death warrant, and that the cup of healing too often foams with *Aqua Tofana?*' 'Poisoning in England', *Saturday review* 1 (1855), pp. 134–5, p. 135.

21 For an overview, see Michael Collins, *Money and banking in the UK: a history* (London: Croom Helm, 1988). For interpretive discussions of the broader social and cultural transformations accompanying these developments, see Boyd Hilton, *The age of atonement: the influence of evangelicalism on social and economic thought, 1795–1865* (Oxford: Oxford University Press, 1988), and G. R. Searle, *Morality and the market in Victorian Britain* (Oxford: Oxford University Press, 1998).

22 There is a growing literature on market morality in the Victorian period. See, in addition to Hilton and Searle, George Robb, *White collar crime in modern England* (Cambridge: Cambridge University Press, 1992), Daniel Itzkowitz, 'Fair enterprise or extravagant speculation: investment, speculation, and gambling in Victorian England', *Victorian studies* 45:1 (2002), pp. 121–47, and Christopher Herbert, 'Filthy lucre: Victorian ideas of money', *Victorian studies* 44:2 (2002), pp. 185–213.

23 David Morier Evans, *Facts, failures and frauds: financial mercantile criminal revelations* (London: Goombridge and Sons, 1859), p. 74.

24 *The Times* (18 June 1856), p. 6. Parliamentary debates in the previous year had developed these themes: the 'system of vicious and improvident speculation' which would follow from limited liability, according to one MP, would 'induce ignorant persons to enter into the most delusive and dangerous undertakings'. *The Times* (27 July 1855), p. 6. The market, according to another, would be littered with companies 'endowed with corporate powers, having no assets and no legal liabilities .. [with] the unlimited power of obtaining credit and entrapping the unwary'. *The Times* (3 August 1855), p. 6.

25 See, e.g. Itzkowitz, 'Fair enterprise or extravagant speculation', p. 122.

26 *The Times* (24 March 1854), p. 8.

27 *Ibid.* (19 October 1854), p. 6.

28 *Ibid.* (24 March 1854), p. 8. For a history of gambling and anti-gaming legislation, see Mark Clapson, *A bit of a flutter: popular gambling and English society, c. 1823–1961* (Manchester: Manchester University Press, 1992).

29 From only a handful at the start of the century, company numbers grew steadily for the first four decades, with 72 new offices established between 1816 and 1844; a further 70 offices were established between 1844 and 1857. The failure rate was also very high: between 1844 and 1857, 108 offices closed. 'Life assurance', *Edinburgh review* 109 (1859), pp. 37–65, pp. 46–7. Barry Supple estimates that there were 150 life insurance offices by early 1850s, and 190 by the mid-1850s. B. Supple, *The Royal Exchange Assurance* (Cambridge: Cambridge University Press, 1970), p. 111. See, in addition to Supple, Geoffrey Clark, 'Life insurance in the society and culture of London, 1700–75', *Urban history* 24:1 (1997), pp. 17–36, and G. Clark, *Betting on lives: the culture of life insurance in England, 1695–1775* (Manchester: Manchester University Press, 1999).

30 Mill, 'Civilization', p. 122. In an influential article challenging Chartist suffrage demands, the noted political essayist and historian Sir Archibald Alison cited life-insurance figures as grounds for rejecting working-class enfranchisement, the preponderance of middle-class policies and the relative absence of working-class policies, he argued, demonstrating that only the former had the disciplined forethought necessary for full citizenship. A. Alison, 'The Chartists and universal suffrage', *Blackwood's Edinburgh magazine* 46 (1839), pp. 289–303, pp. 295–8.

31 *The Times* (10 March 1846), p. 5; 'A chapter on life assurance', *Blackwood's* 74 (1853), pp. 105–16, p. 116, 106. Manuals for insurance brokers urged company representatives to play on this sense of patriarchal duty, and to dwell on the horrors attending the death-bed of the uninsured. See, e.g., J. Baxter Langley, *The life-agent's vade-mecum, and practical guide to success in life assurance business*, 6th edn (London: William Tweedie, 1862), ch. 16.

32 Supple, *The Royal Exchange*, Clark; 'Life insurance'.

33 Robert Vincent, *Life assurance as bearing on social economy* (London: Longman, Brown, Green & Longmans, 1850), p. 19. See also *The ladies' guide to life assurance . . .*, by a lady (London: Partridge, Oakey and Co., 1854), p. 10.

34 'Select Committee on joint stock companies' (1844), cited in Supple, *The Royal Exchange*, p. 116. Contemporary insurance prospectuses highlighted this use: 'borrowers avail themselves of it, as security for the loans they seek; and Lenders, satisfied of its sufficiency, are thereby induced to grant facilities which they would otherwise withhold'. (British and Foreign Life and Fire Assurance Co (London), undated, c. 1830s, in Insurance Box 1, John Johnson Collection, Bodleian Library).

35 *Observations, cautionary and recommendatory, on life assurance* (London:

Green and Co, 1841), p. 4.

36 Cited in Supple, *The Royal Exchange*, pp. 138, 139. This was a concern echoed in contemporary literature, the most notable examples being Dickens's description of the machinations of the Anglo-Bengalese Assurance Company in *The Life and adventures of Martin Chuzzlewit* (1843–44) and Thackeray's indictment of the 'West Diddlesex Fire and Life Insurance Company' in *The Great Hoggerty Diamond* (1849), itself based on a contemporary scandal involving West Middlesex General Annuity Assurance Company.

37 The link between insurance and poisoning did not begin with Palmer: the core murder plot in Lytton's *Lucretia*, for example, involved poisoning for insurance money. Lytton took as his inspiration the case of Thomas Griffiths Wainewright (1839), who was widely suspected of having poisoned his nieces after having insured their lives. Wainewright later provided the inspiration for Dickens's 1859 short story *Hunted down*, in which an insurance agent turns into a detective on the track of a would-be poisoning insurance fraudster. Dickens himself wrote about having visited Wainewright in prison, during which time Wainewright reportedly aligned himself with the market logic of crime, observing: 'Sir, you city men enter on your speculations, and take the chances of them. Some of your speculations succeed, some fail. Mine happens to have failed; yours happens to have succeeded; that is the difference, sir, between my visitor and me'. R. Shelton Mackenzie, *Life of Charles Dickens* (Philadelphia: T. B. Peterson & Brothers, 1870), p. 359.

38 'The crime of the age', *Illustrated times* (2 February 1856), pp. 64–5, p. 64.

39 This is a point nicely developed by Elizabeth Wallace, 'The needs of strangers: friendly societies and insurance societies in late eighteenth-century England', *Eighteenth-century life* 24 (2000), pp. 53–72.

40 'Poison', *Household words* 13 (22 March 1856), 224.

41 There is a large literature on the professionalization of medicine in this period. See especially M. Jeanne Peterson, *The medical profession in mid-Victorian London* (London and Berkeley: University of California Press, 1978) and Anne Digby, *The evolution of British general practice: 1850–1948* (Oxford: Oxford University Press, 1999).

42 On the Anatomy Act, see Ruth Richardson, *Death, dissection and the destitute* (London, Routledge & Kegan Paul, 1988); for sectarianism, see the literature cited in note 73, chapter 2 of the current book.

43 'Criminal poisoning', *Pharmaceutical journal* 15 (1855–6), pp. 289–92, p. 290.

44 For the use of poison in the growing fields of experimental physiology and pharmacology, see John Lesch, *Science and medicine in France* (Cambridge MA and London: Harvard University Press, 1984), especially chs 4–7.

45 'Science in the witness box', *Examiner* (19 January 1856), p. 35.

46 *Ibid.*

47 *Ibid.*

48 *The Times* (24 December 1855), p. 6.

49 'Poisoning in England', *Saturday review* 1 (1855), pp. 134–5, p. 135. At professional meetings medical people could indulge in similar exercises in critical assessment, with one participant going so far as to accuse Taylor of indulgence in a 'transcendentalism of the laboratory'. *Lloyd's weekly London newspaper* (17 February 1856), p. 7.

50 'Doctor in the witness-box', *Dublin University magazine* 47 (1856), pp. 178–95, p. 193.

51 *Illustrated times* (17 May 1856), p. 338. Emphasis original.

52 'The Rugeley suspected poisoning cases', *Lancet* 1 (1856), p. 348. Home Office files show that, guided by Taylor, the Home Office steadfastly refused to provide such information, despite repeated pleas from Palmer's solicitor. PRO HO 45/6260/20–23.

53 'Our interview with Dr Alfred Taylor', *Illustrated times supplement: the Rugeley number* (2 February 1856), p. 91. Emphasis original. At Palmer's trial, Taylor vehemently denied having given Mayhew permission to publish from their discussion, calling it 'the greatest deception that was ever practised on a scientific man; most disgraceful'. *The Queen v. Palmer. Verbatim report of the trial of W. Palmer at the Central Criminal Court, Old Bailey, London, May 14, and following days, 1856 ... Transcribed from the short hand notes of Mr. Angelo Bennett* (London: J. Allen, 1856), p. 147. The Mayhew in question is sometimes identified as Augustus, Henry's brother, but Henry claimed responsibility for the interview in letters to the editors of several leading newspapers.

54 'The doctor in the witness-box', *Dublin University magazine*, p. 194.

55 *Daily telegraph* (15 May 1856), p. 3.

56 *Queen v. Palmer*, p. 24. Cockburn received the backing of Lord Chief Justice Campbell in his closing summation, which acknowledged the common-sense bias against the prosecution's charge of strychnine poisoning, but advised that this had no compelling legal force: 'With respect to the consideration that no strychnia was found in the body, that is for you to consider, and no doubt you will pay great attention to it; but there is no point of law according to which the poison must be found in the body of the deceased; and all that we know respecting the poison not being in the body of Cook is, that in that part of the body that was analysed by Drs. Taylor and Rees they found no strychnia'. (*Ibid.*, p. 319). Having directed the jury on the law, Campbell left this as the central question it had to resolve: 'The question for your consideration is, whether the absence of its detection leads conclusively to the view that this death could not have been caused by the administration of that poison'. (*Ibid.*, p. 325).

57 *Ibid.*, p. 24.

58 Taylor's first edition of *On poisons* provides an overview of the range of tests available at mid-century. Although by the time of Palmer's trial the Belgian chemist Jean Servois Stas had announced a method of isolating absorbed alkaloids, including strychnine, Taylor professed scepticism about its use in

criminal cases, and did not employ it in his analysis of Cook. In reports of the fifteen British pre-Palmer strychnine cases reviewed by Taylor, for example, only six mentioned the use of colour tests. Taylor, 'On poisoning by strychnia, with comments on the medical evidence given at the trial of William Palmer', *Guy's Hospital reports* 2 (3rd ser.) (1856), pp. 269–404, pp. 346–53.

59 *Ibid.*, p. 138.

60 *Ibid.*, p. 152.

61 *Ibid.*, pp. 10–11. Emphasis original.

62 George Knott, *Trial of William Palmer* (Edinburgh and London: William Hodge and Co., 1912), p. 45.

63 *The Queen v. Palmer*, p. 11.

64 *Ibid.*, p. 175.

65 *Ibid.*, pp. 231, 235.

66 *Ibid.*, pp. 197–8.

67 Alternatives to the theory of strychnine poisoning ranged from epileptic convulsions with tetanic complications, angina pectoris, spinal cord irritation of undetermined cause, and tetanic convulsions brought on by wet and cold acting on a body debilitated by syphilis.

68 *Ibid.*, p. 111. Curling, in reply, stated that this was the judgment of a young and comparatively inexperienced practitioner, and that anyway the case in question was not one derived from his own observation. At this stage Cockburn dramatically intervened, claiming to have proof that the case was in fact apocryphal.

69 *Ibid.*, p. 117.

70 *Ibid.*, p. 149.

71 *Ibid.*, pp. 144–5.

72 *Ibid.*, p. 201.

73 See, for example, Thomas Starkie, *Practical treatise on the law of evidence*, 2 vols, 2nd edn (London: J. and W. T. Clarke, 1833), 1, p. 154: 'The testimony of medical men is constantly admitted with respect to the cause of disease or death, . . . as collected from a number of circumstances. Such opinions are admissible in evidence, although the professional witnesses found them entirely on the facts, circumstances, and symptoms established in evidence by others, and without being personally acquainted with the facts'.

74 Robert Christison, 'On the present state of medical evidence', *Edinburgh medical review* 23 (n.s.) (1851), pp. 401–30, pp. 420–1.

75 *Queen v. Palmer*, p. 190. The problematic relationship between author, text, and testimony in fact forms an important subtext running through the trial transcript: questions were posed about whether Taylor and Christison appeared as themselves or as embodiments of their works (e.g. pp. 144 and 200); controversy arose from having textual excerpts read in court in the absence of their still living authors (e.g. pp. 196–7); and the general con-

straints of transcribing experience into writing were discussed at some length (e.g. pp. 201 and 250).

76 *Ibid.*, p. 189.
77 *Ibid.*, p. 148.
78 *Ibid.*, p. 202.
79 *Ibid.*
80 *Ibid.*, p. 174.
81 *Ibid.*, p. 190.
82 *Ibid.*, p. 288. Cockburn's argument received the support of the presiding judge, Lord Chief Justice Campbell who suggested to the jury that while many of Palmer's experts were men of high honour and integrity and scientific knowledge, they might see others as having come forth as 'advocates' (p. 320). For a stimulating analysis of the charges of partisanship among Victorian expert witnesses, see Christopher Hamlin, 'Scientific method and expert witnessing', *Social studies of science* 76 (1986), pp. 485–513.
83 *Queen v. Palmer*, p. 325. Emphasis original.

5

The travails of poison hunting

Interest in Palmer as a case outlived Palmer the man, with his verdict and execution causing almost as much ink to be spilled as his trial had done. The immediate response was a widespread expression of approval, beginning with Campbell's declaration, in passing sentence on Palmer, that he and his fellow justices were 'fully satisfied'. The mainstream press echoed Campbell's sentiment: a *Times* editorial put the weight of informed public opinion squarely behind the decision: 'In the justice of the verdict every one who has followed these memorable proceedings must fully concur'.[1] The professional journals agreed: 'The verdict', the *Law times* opined, 'accords with the public judgment, and with the opinion formed by the gravest and most clamly [*sic*] reflective minds in the Profession, accustomed to weigh the worth of evidence'.[2] From the pages of the medical press, further plaudits rained down on the trial: 'We venture to say that no one accustomed to balance evidence will question the righteousness of the verdict', the *Lancet* wrote, while the *Association medical journal* declared the verdict to be 'without doubt, in accordance with the voice of science and the feeling of the country'.[3] But this was far from the whole story, for the declarations of 'perfect satisfaction' also contained expressions of criticism and often considerable anxiety, about the way the Palmer trial would reflect upon scientific expertise in the courtroom, and how it would be ultimately remembered. Justice had been done, but not without its costs.

Before discussing these underlying concerns, it is worth noting that not even the feeling of the verdict's overall validity was as secure as the editorialists would have had it. In the fortnight between Palmer's conviction and his execution, Palmer's supporters mounted an energetic campaign for a reprieve. The prime organizer was Palmer's solicitor, John Smith, who sent scores of letters to the press and to Whitehall urging intervention in the impending 'legal murder' of his client. Anonymous correspondents and pamphleteers were also busy denouncing the verdict. Members of the scientific community, led by Letheby and Herapath, penned amplifications of the evidence in favour of the convict, while several reports of new chemical experiments claiming to have proven the traceability of minute quantities of strychnine found their way into the public press. Protest culminated in a meeting convened at St Martin's-Hall, Long Acre, on 10 June. The meeting, as reported by a correspondent for *The Times*, was packed, boisterous, and largely supportive, not so much of Palmer as an individual, but of the need for further scrutiny of the scientific evidence that had led to his conviction. The first of the evening's resolutions, moved by Mr. Baxter Langley, called on the Home Secretary, Sir George Grey, to grant a delay of execution in light of the 'grave doubts as to whether or not John Parsons Cook died from strychnia, and it being essential in the interests of society, the progress of science, and the safety of individual life'. In urging passage of the resolution, Langley drew wide applause when he declared that 'if Palmer was executed, he would be executed to satisfy a scientific hypothesis'.[4]

The mainstream press widely condemned these public expressions of support for Palmer as contrary to general, rational opinion, spawned more by maudlin sensibility than by a sense of justice. The most striking and apposite exercise in marginalization appeared in the *Examiner* which, in praising Grey's resistance to these efforts, suggested that the real motive behind much of the Palmerite sentiment was all too well in keeping with the contemporary social ills that Palmer himself typified: 'among those who were not the least anxious to procure his pardon of commutation of punishment', the *Examiner* explained with great indignation, 'were the large number of persons who had bets on his escape from the gallows'.[5] But although the organs of public and professional opinion considered the motive and ultimate justice of the pro-Palmer sentiment suspect at best, they were themselves full of comment, criticism, and suggestions for revising the relationship between science and law as revealed in the Palmer case. While there was no consensus about what had gone wrong, and what needed fixing, it is clear that the universal protestations of enthusiasm for the verdict masked a considerable degree of discomfort.

In the lay press, two main strands emerged in the aftermath of the Palmer conviction to account for the less than ideal light under which scientific evidence had been placed. The first pointed to a basic misunderstanding of the nature and significance of scientific evidence. Editorialists maintained that the amount of attention that had been devoted to the scientific aspects of the case had left the public with an inflated view of the importance of this type of evidence, without, it should be noted, acknowledging their own part in building up these very expectations. Reversing its own earlier professed confidence in toxicology's capacity to make bodies speak, for example, the *Examiner* explained to its readers that expert testimony was not meant to 'prove an entire accusation'. While it was 'next to certain, that without the scientific evidence to make assurance sure, the vilest criminal of our day would have escaped the scaffold', it was not the case – neither should it have been – that science determined the verdict. Experts had simply been asked 'to convert natural into legal certainty; and to take away, from such moral proofs on a matter of less gravity no man would have resisted, the faintest possibility of error. And this they did'.[6]

The *Examiner*, in seeking to instil its readership with a proper sense of perspective on, and confidence in, scientific evidence in criminal trials, significantly revised its own version of how bodies spoke from the grave, and to whom: 'It is important to be widely known, we think, that it is not the chemist alone whom the secret poisoner must now dread. The entire range of medical science is against him'. In place of toxicological reanimation, the body spoke through its symptoms to a corporate medical audience headed by the physiologist. Although chemistry remained 'the chief terror of poisoners', society should recognize and take comfort in the fact that other means of equal evidentiary weight existed: 'Murder that does not cry out of the grave, is yet able to speak (as in this case it did) even by the very form of the death agony'.[7]

Thus, while the imagery of toxicological infallibility required reconsideration in the wake of the Palmer trial, the *Examiner* maintained there was nothing that came out of the trial that should significantly diminish public faith in medico-legal evidence at poisoning cases. A second set of explanations for the weaknesses of science at the Palmer trial, while similarly sparing it as a methodology and a repository of reliable knowledge, was more directly critical of the role of scientists themselves in damaging their public standing. Here the criticism, voiced during the trial itself, was that individual scientists had abandoned the ideal of disinterested science and had become 'dogmatists', 'advocates' of a particular point of view.

Not surprisingly in a climate generally sympathetic to the verdict, it was the defence witnesses whom the press singled out as having betrayed their proper calling. Editorialists offered several distinct but overlapping explanations for the unsatisfactory display made by certain experts. Some highlighted the base motive of financial gain, while others saw the root cause in the more mediated desire for professional self-advancement.[8] Contention was an asset to practitioners toiling at the bottom of a highly competitive field, the *Examiner* explained: 'It will always be observed that if the highest medical authorities are of one opinion, the opposite opinion is sure to be maintained by members of the profession who are of no authority whatever. To maintain a thesis against such a man as Sir Benjamin Brodie, is a distinction for an obscure practitioner . . . It is the cheapest and best advertisement'.[9]

This competitive display of self was magnified in the adversarial courtroom, indeed encouraged, by the machinations of lawyers who 'gloried in medical discord'. Even the most dispassionate and honourable scientific witness, according to a *Lloyd's* editorial, might be drawn in by conditions so uncongenial to the pursuit of scientific truth. The Palmer case had thus left the public with an ambiguous sense of expert credibility. On the one hand, it had demonstrated the attainments of modern medicine and science.

> But, alas, no trial has ever gone so far to prove how prone the highest intellects are to succumb to the promptings of personal vanity, 'that last infirmity of noble minds' . . . Learnedly and wisely and dispassionately, Dr. Taylor, the philosopher and physician, told how and why he believed the man at the bar had done to death the victim of his cupidity. But then the vanity of Dr. Taylor, the man, was touched. And learning and wisdom were forgotten.

If Taylor the scientist had been betrayed by Taylor the man, he was but the noblest victim of the conditions under which he and lesser men had to seek out truth. The ultimate lesson of the Palmer trial, the editorial concluded, was that legal adversarialism, in pitting scientific witnesses against one another 'like rats or prize-fighters', distorted and devalued their evidence: only by protecting scientific evidence from 'cross-examining barristers', *Lloyd's* concluded, could the public recognize 'the purity and brightness of the ore of science untarnished by the dross of poor human vanity'.[10]

Through a variety of strategies, then – by limiting the evidentiary expectations placed on toxicology; by distinguishing between the transcendent interests of science and the possibly contingent motives of its representatives; and by projecting a pure version of expert testimony freed from legal distortion – the lay press in the wake of the Palmer trial by and large sought to bolster the public image of science as a reliable conduit for truth in criminal courts. These discussions also featured in

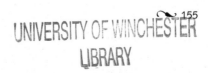

the pages of the medical press, but they were joined by a more funda-mental question about the compatibility of legal and scientific contexts and methods for producing and evaluating evidence. The basic diagnosis of Fleet Street was correct, in the *Lancet*'s view:

> The radical error in all medico-legal affairs is that scientific men are retained for or against the person accused. Instead of appearing in the witness-box as the expounders of science, they appear more in the character of advocates . . . Let a man be ever so honest, what surer method of biasing him can be devised than to pay him a heavy fee, pit him against a scientific opponent holding diametrically opposite opinions, pique his self-love by setting him to prove himself right and everybody else wrong, and, lastly, to stir up his bile with the vexatious cross-questioning and superficial impertinence of men whose peculiarity it is to be vexatious and superficial?[11]

Although lawyerly 'peculiarities' were high-profile targets, the medical critique of the state of scientific evidence saw this as one instance of a wider lack of public appreciation of the true standing of medical evi-dence, both in and out of the courtroom. From within the confines of the trial itself, the machinations of lawyers were successful in part because they could interpose themselves between the pure language of science and the lay jury. The need for translation of scientific evidence opened up a wide field of misunderstanding – whether intentional or not. Even without the 'vexatious and superficial' contribution of legal men, the *Lancet* admitted, the problem of representing medical knowledge to the lay jury was a daunting one:

> It is impossible that science can speak to the unskilled in language so intel-ligible and distinct as she does to her chosen disciples. It could not be expected that twelve men, relying upon their general knowledge and that indefinable, lawless, and treacherous faculty, 'common sense', should esti-mate accurately the value of the medical evidence laid before them. If they sought to be guided by those scientific witnesses whose names carry the greatest weight of authority, they might err; if they committed their judg-ment to the testimony of the greatest number, they might still more proba-bly err; if they sought to unravel the scientific questions before them by the application of their own knowledge and common sense, they were almost sure to err, or to go right only by accident.[12]

Jury verdicts derived from an interpretation of scientific evidence were thus tenuous indeed, but there were grounds for improvement. For the *Lancet*, the solution lay in better public understanding, and in this sense the very problems raised by a case like Palmer's might serve as an opportunity for advancement. The verdict had excited controversy, it argued, because it exposed the gulf between public and scientific notions of proof. 'Juries and the public generally', it explained, 'always look for the material demonstration of the poison in the dead body. They are disposed to overrate the importance of this demonstration, and even to place it before the evidence derived from the observation of the symptoms and the morbid appearances'.[13] This of course echoed one of the central points of evidentiary dispute in the trial itself, but the *Lancet* believed that, if led through the evidence, the public might be persuaded to put aside its materialist bias.

The *Lancet* devoted the better part of its post-trial commentary to beginning precisely this task. Drawing primarily on existing clinical and physiological knowledge of the symptoms of strychnine poisoning, it argued that the case against Palmer could be proven not only without the aid of general evidence, but also without that of chemistry. Signalling the need to rein in the kind of toxicological triumphalism that had marked much of the pre-trial, the *Lancet* concluded its review with the assertion that medicine had 'solved the problem put'. Through the judicious use of instructive opportunities such as this, it added hopefully, 'juries will learn how distinct and independent and authoritative the decision of Medicine may be in cases of this kind; and the public will perceive ample reason for placing firm reliance upon science for the detection and prevention of crime'.[14]

Others amongst the *Lancet*'s medical contemporaries, while sharing its analysis, were less sanguine about the efficacy of education, and looked elsewhere for solutions. The *Association medical journal* was notably more despondent in the aftermath of the trial. Rather than seeking to enlarge the public 'appreciation' of scientific evidence, it conceded failure, and sought excuses in circumstance. Its first leader announcing the verdict set the tone, openly acknowledging the 'scandal' caused by Taylor's inability to find strychnine, and bemoaning Palmer's choice of an agent that had called upon a particularly vulnerable branch of medical knowledge. The *AMJ* looked also to the circumstances of the Cook post-mortem – especially to the fact that Palmer had spilled out the contents of the stomach 'which doubtless contained the unabsorbed dose of strychnine' – to explain the 'failure' of the scientific evidence.

The Palmer debacle, however, ultimately spoke to the need for greater professional solidarity, especially in the pages of the lay press, which had been the site of unseemly partisanship: 'How can we expect the public to respect us, if we will not respect each other – if we will not abstain even from using expressions which do not commonly pass current in the disputes of gentlemen', the *AMJ* demanded in terms befitting its position as the leading voice of medical professionalization. 'It is but rarely that medicine comes prominently before the public; and we ought, therefore, to be specially careful that we do nothing to sully the fair fame of its professors in the eyes of the world: we are afraid, however, that this trial has done more to lower our status than any thing which has occurred within these last twenty years'.[15]

In the courtroom and in the laboratory too, consensus should be actively promoted. Although acceding to the *Lancet*'s bolder assertion that disagreement did not always stem from 'unscientific' considerations, better communication between experts might keep it to a minimum. Had, for example, Herapath and Letheby been let in on the analysis of Cook's fluids, the *AMJ* believed that 'the one doubt which clouds the case would have been set at rest'. This was the way forward, in its view, and in charting out a kind of corporatist expertise it seemed willing to sacrifice individual reputation to the cause. Accordingly, Taylor came out less well in the pages of the *AMJ* than elsewhere, as when his theory of traceless strychnine was used to illustrate the problem of fragmented expertise: 'This is the dictum of a gentleman whose test-tube has brought many a man to the gallows, and it ought, we think, to be corroborated or confuted in a manner as openly as it has been given'.[16] Taylor's failure to find strychnine was a real problem of medical knowledge – not merely one of public perception. It was this sense of uncertainty, regret, and recrimination, that prompted the *AMJ*'s thoroughly unscientific hopes for a gallows confession noted in the introduction to this book. Disappointed in this hope for a secure – if transcendental – solution to the Rugeley poisonings, it urged a re-examination animated by the new spirit of professional solidarity.

Despite broad support for the verdict, then, the Palmer case had raised searching questions about the standing of toxicology as a reliable bulwark against the modern poisoner. Given his position as the virtual embodiment of modern toxicological attainment, coupled with his deep personal involvement in the Palmer trial, it was inevitable that Taylor would enter the fray. In doing so he chose his ground carefully. Refusing to be drawn into ongoing critical correspondence in the daily and medical press, Taylor opted for a vehicle more appropriate to his standing as the nation's leading medico-legal author. In the autumn of 1856, Taylor penned 'On poisoning by strychnia', a fifty-page tract first published in his institutional in-house journal, *Guy's Hospital reports*.[17] Length aside, the form of this article appeared no different from the dozens of earlier communications on toxicological matters that Taylor had published in the *Reports*. However, one only had to look as far as the article's subtitle – in which Palmer's name appears – to understand that this would be devoted to a direct, and often polemical, engagement with contingencies and personalities of the late trial.

Palmer's identity as a medically skilled poisoner provided the basis for 'On poisoning's' core assertion: that the public needed to be re-educated in order to appreciate the testimony delivered at his trial. Through pre-trial press reports, Taylor asserted, the public had been led to believe in an inflated doctrine of toxicological materialism – that 'no man can die of poison except poison be found in his body, and that unless the material instrument of death be *always*, and *under all circumstances*, forthcoming, upon such charges, no man's life would be safe!' What these reports had 'studiously concealed', however, was that

> to men of craft and skill in the medical profession, deadly poisons are accessible, which may destroy life in such doses and under such modes of administration, that, while no chemical tests can reveal their presence in the body, their unlawful use may be surely and satisfactorily indicated ... by the symptoms which they produce.[18]

Ordinary expectations of chemical demonstration, in cases of special sophistication like this one, had to be laid aside, with the clinical acumen of the physician taking a lead role in adducing proof of poisoning.

The special circumstances of the Palmer case, then, turned Taylor's negative analytical results into tokens of his credibility as an expert, rather than his fallibility. By contrast, his critics' claims of toxicological infallibility marked them out as enthusiasts, their professed ability to detect minute quantities of strychnine attributable not to their keener analytical skill but to their willingness to place 'bold reliance ... upon infinitesimal results'.[19] Taylor's criticism of his (frequently named) critics, then, put into focus the potential for toxicological plasticity, the possibility that analytical indicators from the laboratory could be differently interpreted – could exist not as plain fact but, in a charge repeatedly invoked by Taylor, as products of an unreliable analytical imagination.

In making this claim, Taylor's text spelled out the elements that might lead the analyst into error. Chemical tests, Taylor asserted, involved judgment and interpretation, and thus evidence derived from them entailed a subjective element. He illustrated this point by invoking that most slippery of toxicological signs – colour:

> The chemist demonstrates, as he says, by certain colours, the presence in the dead body of the fifty thousandth or the twenty thousandth of a grain of poison; one of a sanguine temperament will tell you that, beyond all doubt, it is strychnia; a second will affirm that the appearance is equivocal; and a third will tell out that he disbelieves altogether that it indicates the presence of the poison'.[20]

The declaration made by Taylor and Rees that they had not found strychnine in Cook's body thus constituted a principled resistance to toxicological over-interpretation: 'although we obtained, in this instance, by the use of the tests, certain changes of colour, which an ardent imagination might, I believe, have easily construed into proofs of the presence of strychnine, we declined to take this view'.[21]

Taylor pressed this point further, paradoxically, by engaging in an extended passage of pure fiction, which lays out the hostile interrogation he would have faced had he 'taken a more sanguine view of this matter'. In it the conjured defence attorney tears into the claims of strychnine detection based on 'a blue, purple, and red colour, upon adding to some sort of extract obtained from the dead body'. He opens up the toxicologist's tool-kit, finding numerous sources of potential error: one of the reagents used was itself strongly coloured, for example, while another produced a similar colour with numerous organic substances besides the one tested for. 'I have a great respect for science', the interrogator declares, 'but when I find two witnesses thus coming forward to swear away a man's life upon the 100th, aye, the 1000th of a grain of something which they suppose to be strychnia, just because they noticed a little flickering blue and purple colour when they added their chemicals to it, I cannot suppress my indignation'.[22]

Taylor resumed his efforts to stabilize the Palmer case, and to exorcize the spectre of toxicological enthusiasm, when in early 1859 he produced the second edition of his textbook, *On poisons*. As might be expected in a work ostensibly devoted to delivering a consensual version of best practice, its tone is more measured than the 1856 tract, but its objectives are nonetheless clear. 'In nearly every chapter on every poison in this volume', Taylor observes, 'the reader will find that chemistry has in some cases completely failed to reveal the presence of poison, while in others it has misled an "expert" to swear to the presence of poison in a definite quantity in a dead body when the whole was a fiction of the imagination'.[23] And though Taylor makes an attempt to translate his critique into the terms of abstract toxicological truth, Palmer's role in framing his arguments cannot be disguised, Taylor himself noting in several places the unusual degree to which the case (described in one place as 'that memorable case which has furnished some point of illustration to almost every department of medical jurisprudence') is invoked in, and indeed shapes, the text.[24]

To see how Taylor's involvement in the Palmer case affected his presentation of the general principles of toxicology, we can consider how the two issues highlighted from 'On poisoning' – the validity of convictions without chemical evidence, and the potential for subjective distortion of analytical results – are differently treated in the 1848 and 1859 editions of *On poisons*. Although the 1848 text acknowledged that toxicology might fail to deliver tangible proof, it did not devote much attention to developing the point. Taylor explains that many poisons could not as yet be detected, and that those poisons which were capable of chemical demonstration might, under certain largely unspecified circumstances, resist chemical analysis. He illustrates the viability of convictions without chemical evidence by reference to a few legal precedents, starting with a foundation of dubious solidity – Donnellan's controversial conviction on the evidence provided by Lady Boughton's sense of smell. Acknowledging the objections raised against this conviction, Taylor adds two further examples: a Scottish case from 1821, and an Irish one twenty years later. Taylor here concludes this unremarkable discussion, turning instead to the reasons why the public and legal officers preferred chemical evidence to the fallible criteria of symptoms and post-mortem appearances.[25]

Taylor's 1859 account of the limits of chemical evidence, by contrast, is nearly doubled in length – the extra pages almost entirely accounted for by comments on Palmer. It begins almost exactly as described above, with the sole addition of a French case of a medical poisoner to supplement the Scottish and Irish precedents. After this, however, Palmer takes over. The primary purpose of the inserted exposition is to emphasize the importance of proofs other than chemical. To insist on the extraction of poison 'in a visible and tangible form', he observes, 'would be casting aside physiology and pathology, and requiring our law-authorities to place entire and exclusive confidence in the crucible and the test-tube of the chemist'.[26] Taylor disrupts the first edition's explanation as to why the public and law authorities favoured chemical demonstration by inserting, after his observation about clinical and post-mortem limitations, a new declaration: 'Chemists, however, are not infallible, and instances might be adduced of their swearing in the most positive manner to the presence of poison in cases in which they have been afterwards obliged to admit that none existed!'[27]

In an expanded section on 'fallacies in chemical analysis', which concludes the chapter, Taylor turns to the topic of colour tests. Here he supplements the 1848 edition's previously abstract discussion of the dangers of underdetermination (that indicators resulting from chemical tests might apply to more than one substance), by reference to the over-reliance on colour for the detection of alkaloids like strychnine.[28] 'The mere indications of colour', he asserts, 'although they may give rise to suspicion, cannot be relied on as conclusive evidence'. But Taylor then extends his remarks beyond the tests for elusive alkaloids to a more general statement on the inherent dangers of analysis based on indicators that lend themselves to divergent interpretation. Citing the French chemist Alphonse Devergie's dictum about the deceitfulness of colour testing, Taylor concludes by observing that 'four persons may look at the same coloured product, and it will be found to present to each a different shade or tint'.[29]

Here, as in numerous other places in the 1859 edition, Taylor is attempting several things at once. He wishes to defend his evidence in the Palmer case – most especially his alleged 'failure' to find strychnine in Cook's body – against ongoing criticism led by Herapath and Letheby. In this effort his strategy is to marginalize them as enthusiasts with an overly developed sense of imagination. To accomplish this, Taylor is constrained to take toxicology out of the realm of abstract, disembodied science, and to cast it as an activity with a potentially subjective and embodied component. This is not his final purpose, of course – toxicology, ideally, *should* be abstract and disembodied, but only after it has been purged of the distortions which the Palmer case had done so much to make manifest. In his battle against enthusiasm, in other words, Taylor was led to emphasize the limits of chemical analysis in order to better cast it as credible science. But this was a difficult balance to maintain, with the boundaries of his critique of toxicological excess always threatening to spill over into more generalizable observations on the nature of toxicological evidence itself. Taylor could not, for example, stress over-reliance on infinitesimal test-tube results without raising the relative importance of clinical and post-mortem evidence – that is, advertising the test-tube's lack of independent declarative force. Neither could he emphasize the misinterpretability of colour tests without opening up the toxicologist's lab to the kind of experimental regress that he and other toxicologists had blamed the adversarial courtroom for inciting.

The 1859 edition of *On poisons*, in this sense, was an intermediary product, designed to address the distortions head on, but not to reify them as a necessary feature of toxicological work. The intended trajectory of Taylor's reconfiguration of toxicology can be discerned in the third edition of his work, published in 1875. In this edition, Taylor's polemic had been translated into a calmer statement of toxicological truths. Over half of the direct references to Palmer were cut, and the lessons learned from it were presented more as abstract principles than contingent claims.[30] With erasure came the semblance of objectified knowledge derived from the case – the case in this instance being fully integrated as a general set of toxicological principles. Moreover, the second edition's emphasis on toxicological limits, although not eliminated, was radically curtailed. Most significantly, the whole section on 'fallacies in chemical analysis', which had served as a culmination of the second edition's defence of non-detection, was dropped from the third edition. Thus, Taylor's remarks about the dangers of relying on subjective indicators like colour – which were necessary in explaining his own testimony in the wake of Palmer, but which equally called attention to the embodied nature of toxicological evidence as a matter of general principle – were nowhere to be found.

The contrast between the 1859 and 1875 editions of *On poisons* shows how Taylor might use his position as textbook author to codify Palmer as a stable 'case', and to recoup some of the ground ceded to toxicological scepticism by his explicit criticism of the distorted toxicological imagination. But between the two editions Taylor found himself embroiled in another controversial case that, in conjunction with the questions raised by the Palmer trial, made his capacity to embody authoritative detachment deeply problematic. No sooner had the ink dried on his 1859 text, than Taylor's reputation, and by extension the reputation of toxicological expertise itself, was thrown into deeper confusion by another alleged poisoning doctor.

At the centre of the Thomas Smethurst case stood another doctor whose respectable façade masked a sensational reality. The essential background is as follows: born in 1811, Thomas Smethurst was a self-styled surgeon who for years had worked in various fields of alternative medicine, including a stint in charge of a Surrey hydrotherapy clinic.[31] He ceased practising in the early 1850s, and settled in London lodgings with his wife, who was some twenty years his senior. In 1858 he began an affair with a fellow lodger, Isabella Bankes, a woman in her forties and of independent means. Smethurst left his wife in December, and entered into a bigamous marriage with Bankes. Within a few months of becoming the new Mrs Smethurst, Bankes fell ill with diarrhoea, vomiting, and fever. She was seen by three doctors over a period of roughly a month, but her case resisted medical treatment, and attendants begin to suspect something was interfering with their remedies. During the course of her illness, one of these attendants asked Smethurst for samples of her evacuations for examination, and Smethurst duly complied. These were then referred to Taylor while Bankes was still alive, and his preliminary analysis indicated the presence of a metallic deposit, which he suspected was either arsenic or antimony. On 2 May 1859, one day before Bankes's death, Smethurst was apprehended on magistrate's warrant for attempted poisoning.

At the subsequent magistrate's hearings, witnesses attending the post-mortem investigation testified that Bankes's corpse revealed the presence of inflammation, but no clear traces of mineral poison.[32] Taylor was called to testify to the results of analyses undertaken by himself with the assistance of his Guy's colleague, William Odling. Despite Taylor's earlier discovery of a metallic deposit (which he now identified as arsenic) in one of Bankes's sick-bed evacuations, their analysis of the viscera and other materials sent after post-mortem revealed no indications of poison. Analysis of Smethurst's extensive collection of medicines also yielded nothing, with one exception: in 'bottle number 21', Taylor deposed that he and Odling had discovered arsenic, but through unconventional means.

They had submitted a portion of the liquid contained in this bottle to the Reinsch process for isolating arsenic. This process was developed in 1841 by the German chemist Hugo Reinsch, who proclaimed it a safer and simpler test than Marsh's. Among its improvements, Reinsch and his supporters urged, was that it eliminated a source of possible contamination by dispensing with zinc as its core testing material. Reinsch's alternative process involved the introduction of pure and highly polished copper gauze into the suspect liquid mixed with hydrochloric acid. If arsenic were present, it would combine with the acid to form a gas and leave a greyish film on the copper. Taylor, citing its relative ease and greater conditions of purity, had become an early convert to the Reinsch process, and by the time of the Smethurst trial had been using it as a key instrument in his hunt for arsenic for almost two decades. Taylor was much surprised, however, by his application of the Reinsch test to the contents of bottle 21. When the copper gauze was introduced, the liquid in the bottle rapidly dissolved it. In response, Taylor and Odling took the unusual step of introducing more and more copper gauze into the liquid, until its capacity to dissolve the copper was finally exhausted. At this point, when they introduced a fresh copper gauze, it 'at once received the arsenic'.[33]

Taylor explained this unusual analytical sequence to the magistrate's court as follows: bottle 21, he asserted, contained a combination of chlorate of potash and arsenic. Chlorate of potash was an 'innocent medicine': a diuretic used to 'purify the system from all noxious matter'. He had never in his experience met with it in combination with a mineral poison like arsenic, and neither was there any legitimate medical rationale for the combination. There was, Taylor suggested, a sinister rationale for the potion's presence amongst Smethurst's stock of medicines: chlorate of potash would have the effect of speeding the absorption and elimination of arsenic from the body, thus intensifying the effects of small doses of arsenic and making it difficult to detect post-mortem. In this respect, the absence of arsenic in the body of Bankes (which, unlike strychnine in the Palmer case, *ought* to have been detectable if administered) was entirely explicable – Bankes had been slowly, scientifically, poisoned with arsenic.[34]

Smethurst was charged with Bankes's murder and remanded for trial, but in the meantime Taylor continued to labour over the contents of bottle 21, apparently troubled by the unexpected reaction of its contents to Reinsch's process. The solution to the puzzle, according to the testimony brought out at the subsequent trial, was proposed by the veteran chemist William Brande. The arsenic detected by Taylor, Brande suggested, had been deposited into the solution by impurities contained in the copper gauze.[35] The possibility of copper contamination in the Reinsch process, Brande and Taylor asserted during the trial, was an entirely new idea in chemistry. While it was well known that arsenic was an impurity in raw copper, it had also been assumed that the process of refinement, which involved extensive exposure to heat, eliminated any trace of the volatile metal. His analytical results, as Taylor later insisted, had thus exposed a 'latent fallacy', in the process, 'the existence of which neither Reinsch nor any toxicologist of repute had had, up to that date, the slightest suspicion'.[36] Yet the plain fact remained: by feeding tainted copper into the liquid to 'exhaust' its dissolving powers, Taylor had himself introduced the arsenic that he subsequently detected.

Once convinced of his mistake, Taylor informed those charged with the conduct of the case, who decided nonetheless to proceed to trial. In its opening statement, the prosecution acknowledged Taylor's error, but held that his initial discovery of arsenic in Bankes's evacuation was sufficient grounds on which to build a case. The presiding judge lent support to this claim, advising the jury that while Taylor's mistake should be taken into account, it was in itself no reason to impugn the entire testimony of so eminent a practitioner. The defence, however, unsurprisingly argued that Taylor's adventures in the laboratory rendered his other chemical evidence invalid. Revising Taylor's published criticisms of analytical over-indulgences, Smethurst's lead attorney insisted that the idea that a crime had been committed itself rested on a 'stupid' theory of subtle poisoning – 'merely the offspring of a fertile brain' – that was conjured up to account for the absence of any poison in the body of the deceased.[37]

There is no need to enter into a detailed analysis of the arguments adduced at the trial. Suffice it to say that on 19 August, the fifth day of his trial, the jury convicted Smethurst. The verdict generated an immediate storm of protest, with petitions sent to the Home Office signed by thousands, including special petitions sent by medical practitioners throughout the country.[38] The Home Office responded to the deluge by announcing a review of the case, to be conducted by the eminent physician (and prosecution witness in the Palmer case), Sir Benjamin Brodie. For several weeks between the verdict and the final decision to reprieve Smethurst, the debate on the case was intense.

Unlike the Palmer case, in which the balance of opinion, whatever lingering concern there might have been about the absence of detected strychnine, upheld the conviction and the death sentence imposed, the majority of editorials and letters generated in the wake of the Smethurst case urged that the flaws in the scientific evidence necessitated a reconsideration of the verdict. Taylor's frank admission of error in his search for that most common and ostensibly traceable of all poisons, arsenic, featured prominently in these arguments, representing for them at once a practical and symbolic violation of modern toxicological order. The toxicologist who generated poison through his own processes, clearly, raised questions about his command over the material and technical elements of his presumed expertise. The *British medical journal* observed that Taylor's actions had raised inevitable, and legitimate, questions about laboratory practice: 'what guarantee have we that some fatal error has not been made in the course of his long distillations? that his tests are pure? ... If test-tubes and wire-gauze are to be the fatal instruments of justice, the public should at least be convinced that no error has arisen in their application'.[39] *Lloyd's* put the case against Taylor more directly, warning of the consequences of such 'bungling' evidence: 'The introduction of scientific evidence in trials for murder is indeed dangerous, when dirty testing materials may liberate poison, and convict an innocent man'.[40]

Taylor's practical violation of toxicological purity, many commentators observed, was matched by an analogous conceptual violation. Following the lead of Smethurst's attorney, they suggested that Taylor had been led into error through his own imaginative excesses. He had squared the difficulties in his analytical results, the *Lancet* lamented, by recourse to an explanation better suited to historical fiction than scientific fact. In his initial testimony before the magistrates, Taylor had imputed to Smethurst a 'diabolical ingenuity' that enabled him to create a subtle, slow poison: 'the chlorate of potash, which is one of the most innocent materials for lotions and saline draughts to be met with in the Pharmacopoeia, was stigmatized as something horrible, and Smethurst was compared to the Borgias, for acuteness and fiendish cunning as a poisoner'. If not checked, the *Lancet* continued, such speculative evidence threatened to negate recent progress in poison detection: 'an infinitesimal toxicology might, in the present day, become almost as dangerous as the accusations of witchcraft in the fifteenth century'. The *BMJ* was in complete agreement: if nothing were done to address the problem, 'the horrors which flourished in the days of witchcraft, when human life hung upon the lips of any old crone, will be but too faithfully represented by the horrors which will flow from the pseudo-scientific evidence of the present day'.[41]

Some four weeks following his conviction, Smethurst was reprieved – a result broadly welcomed by commentators in the lay press.[42] Medical journals, although similarly supportive of the outcome, were dismayed at the way that the Home Office publicly justified its decision to grant Smethurst a free pardon. This radical step had been necessary, the Home Secretary announced, 'not from any defect in the constitution or proceedings of our criminal tribunals, but from the imperfection of medical science, and from the fallibility of judgment, in an obscure malady, even of skilful and experienced medical practitioners'.[43] This slur on medical and scientific evidence in general was greeted with outrage, nowhere more intense than in the editorial pages of the *Lancet*. Rehearsing the well-entrenched science/law opposition, the *Lancet* blamed the errors made at the trial on the fact that expert witnesses had laboured 'under artificial restrictions invented by lawyers, which are calculated to impede the discovery of scientific truth'. 'Justice ties her bandage over the eyes of Science', it complained, 'and then calls upon Science to declare what she sees!' It was, in fact, in the 'second trial' of Smethurst evidence – the one conducted through free debate between men of science, presided over by one of its leading lights, and aired in the pages of a free professional and lay press – that these artificial restrictions had been overcome. Through this process it had become clear that whatever blame accrued to the expert evidence lay not with science itself, but with the fallible judgment of individuals called to represent it: 'If a chemist discover arsenic where it does not exist', it pointedly demanded, 'shall he therefore blame the imperfection of Science?' Since the trial, it concluded hopefully, 'Science has spoken out distinctly enough; she has amply exposed the fallacies of individuals, and vindicated her own capacity'.[44]

The *Lancet* thus put a brave face on the Smethurst episode: even if the leading representative of toxicology needed to be sacrificed in this case, this did not necessarily nullify his expertise generally, and neither, more emphatically still, did it constitute a stain on the science that he represented. Yet it was impossible to ignore the climate of scepticism that had descended upon the toxicological project in the wake of the recent controversies. Citing the Palmer and Smethurst cases as prime causes, a correspondent to the *Chemical news* declared that 'at present, it must be confessed, neither the judge, the jury, nor the public, have any confidence in the scientific evidence in cases of poisoning'.[45] *The Times* bemoaned the fact that modern criminal poisoning had made toxicology in turn so exposed to failure: in cases of subtle poisoning, it lamented, we must 'pin our faith upon the conclusions of chymists, and hang a fellow-creature because a small crystal, so minute that it can only be recognized by the microscope, is exhibited on a scrap of copper wire'.[46]

Taylor's own response to the Smethurst case seemed to confirm this sense of unease about the project with which he had long been associated. This can be discerned in the differences in content and especially in tone between his published defence of the Smethurst evidence and that written three years earlier in the wake of the Palmer trial. Again using *Guy's Hospital reports* as his outlet, Taylor issued, in the guise of a comprehensive overview of the 'Facts and fallacies connected with the research for arsenic and antimony', a lengthy commentary on the Smethurst trial.[47] Taylor rose to the challenge, using the opportunity to uphold the integrity of his discovery of poison in the evacuations, to criticize the *ex post facto* 'sagacity' of his critics by showing how they too might have fallen into error, and to insist that the latent fallacy in the Reinsch process, now that it had been discovered, was easy to avoid.

But Taylor's defence was noticeably less robust than his earlier effort, overshadowed by an implicit admission that he had made the job of toxicologists, for the foreseeable future, much more complicated. However secure the Reinsch test might be in the hands of the watchful toxicologist, its reputation was not so easily recouped: 'There is no reason to believe that the use of ordinary copper is attended with any risk in the employment of Reinsch's process, merely because it contains traces of arsenic in intimate chemical union', he insisted. Yet 'it may be a question whether, out of deference to public opinion, a substance containing arsenic in any form, or in any proportion, should be used for the detection and separation of this poison'.[48] Public opinion, a perennial concern for the toxicologist, here takes on a newly dominant role. In the wake of the Smethurst case, Taylor seemed resigned to ceding control of the testing process to an open-ended and newly invigorated public scepticism:

> The only plan now open to an analyst is, to seek for the purest articles which he can obtain, and to test their purity by every conceivable method before he resorts to their use. If he desires to escape the censure of the public, and the uncharitable criticisms of some fellow-labourers in the same branch of research, he must go beyond the ordinary routine of testing his materials. He must look for substances, the presence of which they have hitherto ignored or disregarded; or, in the end, some of them will be found to claim credit, however unjustly, for a degree of caution which they have themselves never exercised.[49]

However, there was a real danger that toxicology could not sustain itself in such a critical environment: that it would prove vulnerable to those who would take advantage of the toxicologist's open-ended search for lurking fallacies to thwart even properly constituted chemical evidence. Toxicology's enemies, Taylor mournfully concluded, 'may for a time succeed in their object'.[50]

Taylor's apprehensions proved not unfounded. As far as his own reputation was concerned, although he continued to be consulted as an authority on matters relating to poison, he never again reached the oracular status that many had attributed to him in the build-up to the Palmer trial. Indeed, the very cornerstone of his claim to inhabit the voice of objective authority came under increasing scrutiny. In the immediate aftermath of the Smethurst case, the *BMJ*, condemning the 'farce' of divided toxicological expertise, singled out Taylor's use of his authorial position to fight his corner for special criticism: 'throughout his ample volume *On poisons*', it lamented, he 'never allows an opportunity to escape of sneering at the scientific attainments' of Herapath and Letheby, leading the public to wonder in desperation whether there was something intrinsic in 'poison-hunting which breeds these unnatural storms in regions where the calm atmosphere of science should alone prevail'.[51] This critique persisted, moreover, beyond the heated atmosphere of the Smethurst debacle. In an otherwise favourable review of the 1865 edition of Taylor's general textbook, *Principles and practice of medical jurisprudence*, the *Lancet* declared itself 'pained to see how Dr Taylor makes use of his position as writer of an admirable and authoritative handbook to pillory experts who have been opposed to him in various cases; . . . Even if Dr Taylor had never on any occasion tripped in his evidence', it added pointedly, 'it would be ungenerous to avenge himself in his handbook on the experts who were opposed to him in Court'.[52]

Taylor's difficulties in the courtroom led others to question the very foundational claims upon which he and others had staked the social value of modern toxicology – that it served as an essential bulwark against the growing and commonly underestimated threat of secret poisoning. Following Taylor's reiteration of this claim in an 1862 poisoning trial, the essayist W. S. Austin drew attention to his words, not in order to urge greater social vigilance, but to suggest that Taylor's perception had become distorted. If the charge were true, Austin continued in a way that mirrored the well-established discourse of secret poisoning that had been circulating more or less unchallenged in prior decades, 'we have, as a nation, sadly degenerated since the early part of the seventeenth century'. Yet he believed there was reason to resist Taylor's claims as grounded less in fact than his 'enthusiasm' for his sphere of expertise, an enthusiasm 'which blinds his judgment and weakens his logical power. In one sense', he pointedly concluded, 'much erudition makes him mad'.[53] Some years later, even the *Times* editorialists, who in earlier decades had instructed readers about the real dangers of undetected secret poisoning, offered a similar diagnosis. Taylor's insistence on the poison threat marked him as 'one of those scientific monomaniacs, not uncommon in his profession, who dwell so much upon one subject or theory, to the exclusion of all others, that at last it fairly possesses and runs away with them'.[54]

At the start of the 1850s, Robert Christison had written of the great confidence invested in modern toxicological evidence. Given its capacity to deliver authoritative judgments about the facts of poisoning, Christison had declared, 'it is now no uncommon thing for the prisoner's counsel to admit that part of the case altogether, and to look in quite another direction for the chance of a successful defence'.[55] It was a debatable claim in 1851, but by the end of the decade it would have seemed little short of preposterous, as commentators took note of experts' recent difficulties at poisoning trials, and the seemingly endless opportunities for challenging their evidence. The controversies of the 1850s provided dramatic evidence of a number of connected problems: of biased and self-interested advocacy masquerading as objective expertise; and of disagreement amongst experts about the proper form and scope of toxicological evidence, disagreements fuelled by adversarial courtroom procedures and the interposition of individual toxicologists' unreliable imaginations. Toxicologists, *The Times* lamented in the wake of the Smethurst trial, 'apply their tests, and report from the secret chambers of nature, like interpreters of an unknown tongue; but the interpreters of nature do not agree. The tests themselves require tests, and create fresh questions as to their own action'.[56]

Concerns of this kind fed directly into a growing debate taking shape from the early 1860s onwards about the need to restructure the relationship between expert evidence and law. This debate, conducted in the pages of the lay, legal, and medical press, and at professional venues like the British Association for the Advancement of Science, the Society of Arts, the Social Science Association, the Juridical Society, and the Law Amendment Society, spawned a host of proposals aimed at moving away from the contentious, individualist, and potentially interested image of expertise, and towards a model in which science could speak with a unified, stable voice.[57] Toxicological experts, according to one such plan, should conduct their analyses on a collective rather than an individual basis. This would enable them to 'watch each other, and thereby watch for the accused person', in the view of the *BMJ*, which added hopefully that under these conditions 'we should have no disputes in court about impure tests; and the finding would silence the cavils of mere outsiders, anxious to hear their own voices'.[58] Others went further, suggesting that this corporate expertise might be granted official recognition, a status comparable to the continental model of court appointed experts. Despite its statist overtones, the *Lancet* gave qualified backing to this plan in cases of 'special difficulty', arguing that evidence by official committee compared favourably with native practice, which involved 'leaving the matter to one individual, who implicitly believes the faintest reactions he can obtain in his laboratory'.[59] A cognate plan sought recognition not for experts themselves, but for the protocols they were to follow. 'What is wanted is a general scheme for a complete examination of any suspected matters *for all known poisons*', the *Chemical news* ventured, adding that government should provide the funds for such a venture: 'we have Toxicologists who could supply us with this, if they had any inducement to devote the time and labour which would be required'.[60]

Suggestions for reforming the selection of experts and their practices were matched by those aimed at transforming the context in which they appeared, largely by protecting the experts from legal adversarialism. Many argued that scientific assessors attached to the court, sitting in an advisory capacity for the benefit of the judge and jury and charged with the examination of expert witnesses, were the proper means of turning the courtroom into a space conducive to delivering consensual scientific evidence. The Manchester chemist Robert Angus Smith, in a seminal address delivered at the Society of Arts in January 1860, urged still further protection, arguing that the expert witness should be allowed to deliver his evidence in written form. Currently, Smith complained, 'his careful elaboration of the subject is made into a rough mixture of thoughts; he weighed his words carefully at home, and wrote his evidence patiently and with scrupulous attention to exact phraseology, and now he finds that the great and the small are confounded together by the extreme skill of the practised examiner'.[61]

Debates about proposals such as these, it should be noted, were concerned with more than poisoning trials. Although the Palmer and Smethurst cases were often explicitly cited as reference points, discussions also encompassed parallel criticisms about the conflicting and seemingly self-interested expert testimony increasingly on display in civil courts and in parliamentary hearings (e.g. in patent cases and suits over water purity and other environmental nuisances), as well as in other medico-legal disputes – notably insanity cases. At their root, Christopher Hamlin argues, were fundamental issues about the place of science in modern society: was science a dispassionate, disinterested pursuit of objective truth by a community of consensual practitioners, or a more contingent, applied activity, one seeking not transcendent truth but practical, and disputable, results for particular markets? According to the former view, expert disagreements at criminal trials were highly visible – and damaging – signs that science was being corrupted. But, according to the latter, courtroom disputes were not pathological in themselves. Indeed, expert adversarialism might serve to advance the cause of science, by encouraging explorations of an unconventional but potentially fruitful nature.[62]

But this wider context does not diminish the significance of what in these plans was specific to the story of toxicology that has been developed over the course of this book. Proposals to establish a collective voice of expertise spoke directly to the ills that seemingly beset Victorian toxicology: monomania, the unnatural storms of poison-hunters, the interpretive plasticity of their evidence. In the context of poisoning trials, it was the toxicologist, as much as any other courtroom figure, who was targeted for restraint.

These sober assessments constituted an important framework for reconceptualizing poison and its detection in the aftermath of the controversies of the 1850s, with the scientific difficulties inherent in poisoning trials continuing to serve as a touchstone for plans to reform expert evidence. Despite decades of discussion and numerous attempts to frame appropriate legislation, however, these proposals were never fully implemented.[63] Several reasons might account for this: the failure, in practice, of informal exercises in collective expertise,[64] and the difficulty of constructing and agreeing official standards of proof, for example. At the end of the century the *Lancet* lamented that even in the most developed sub-field of toxicology – the detection of arsenic – experts continued to disagree over proper procedures: 'Some chemists are in favour of one method and some in favour of another, fallacies are pointed out in methods previously held to be exact, and discarded methods have come to the front again, being, as it is asserted, made more accurate by some modification in detail'.[65]

At a broader level, proposals for officially sanctioned expertise and court-appointed scientific advisers ran up against deeply entrenched commitments to adversarialism and jury independence as bulwarks of English liberties. In a much-cited review of reform proposals in the aftermath of the Smethurst case, the noted jurist James Fitzjames Stephen told the Judicial Society in November 1859 that calls for expert assessors represented a misguided and 'timid anxiety to divide responsibility'.[66] Jury verdicts, Stephen explained, were properly based not on demonstrable truth but on belief beyond reasonable doubt, and thus operated according to historically grounded common sense rather than cutting-edge science. Although Stephen could appreciate the appeal of expert assessors in those 'very exceptional cases in which the evidence is of so refined a nature as to leave a substantial doubt on the minds of men of ordinary intelligence', he nonetheless doubted 'whether convictions, so obtained, would or ought to give satisfaction to the public at large'.[67] On these grounds, Stephen concluded, 'the most ancient and most popular institution in the country should be let alone'.[68]

There are deeper considerations, however, that help in understanding why attempts to impose a regime of restraint on the treatment of scientific evidence proved problematic in the specific case of criminal poisoning trials. As this book has argued throughout, poison could not be fully contained within a framework of rational procedures. Poison spoke essentially to imaginations, anchored in public and scientific conceptions of history, crime, and the body, and toxicology was inescapably embedded in this network of associations. It was this characteristic that lent poison trials their extraordinary resonance: as an 1864 article appearing in *Blackwood's Edinburgh magazine* observed, a poison case was an occasion of rare anticipation, 'something that is to be two-thirds emotional and one-third scientific – where the interest vacillates between the most powerful passions and the pangs of arsenic; and the listener is alternately carried from the domestic hearth to the laboratory and back again'.[69] No expert assessor or committee of consensual toxicologists could expect to contain such a dynamic convergence.

The end of this story, then, is *not* that the crime of poisoning lost its capacity to fascinate. Far from it – for the remainder of the century, each decade produced its own celebrated poison trials that in their own ways commanded wide scientific and public attention. What does seem to have changed in light of the experience of toxicology in the 1850s, however, was the sense of heroic urgency of the battle between the modern, civilized, scientific poisoner, and his mirror opposite. Criminal poisoning, self-consciously built up in public discourse over the previous decades as the 'crime of civilisation', after its apogee in the 1850s lost much of its coherence as a pressing cause for concern. As far as toxicology was concerned, the limits dramatized by the Palmer and Smethurst cases suggested the need to retreat into a more reflexive position: evidence by committee, defensive monitoring of its own procedures and claims, deferral to public scepticism. But if one were to look for the continuation of the emotive force of poison in the following few decades, it would be best to turn not to the popular or scientific press, but to places where the relationship between fact and imagination was less fraught with practical difficulties. In the literary realm, the problems encountered in the making of a modern toxicology received a new articulation, in a framework which, while retaining the compelling interest of a real poison case, might better re-work, and possibly contain, its problematic elements.

For our purposes, there can be no one better to represent this migration than Charles Dickens. Over the preceding pages Dickens has appeared as an interested observer of the world of Victorian poison, and it therefore comes as no surprise that he responded directly to both the Palmer and Smethurst trials. His weekly magazine, *Household words*, carried several Palmer-related entries, including an article on the toxicology of strychnine, and an attempt to reconcile Palmer's self-possessed demeanour during and after his trial with the justice of his conviction.[70]

Dickens's reaction to Smethurst's reprieve was marked by a savage satire on its implications for criminal law, criticizing trial by popular opinion and the press and the subversion of credible scientific evidence by a combination of legal perversion and the willingness of experts to indulge in gratuitous contention.[71] In these and other contributions to *Household words* and its successor *All the year round*, Dickens showed himself largely sympathetic to the travails of toxicological expertise. Indeed, Dickens could use the freedoms of fiction to press the case for toxicology more fervently than could its own representatives.

In December 1862, Dickens, in his capacity as 'convenor' of *All the year round*, introduced his readers to 'The modern alchemist'. Framed as an encounter between the magazine's correspondent and the twelfth-century alchemist Artephius, the article is a deliberate and sustained amalgam of fact and fantasy. It begins on an indeterminate note: the correspondent, whilst reading Artephius's alchemical text, experiences a vision of the ancient author, a vision whose reality he immediately questions: 'Have I lost my wits in study of your secret book, O master of the innermost of man? Was it true, or did it only seem to me, that at the ninth hour of the ninth day of the month Nine, or November, the book rose as I read in it, the parchment cover of my Artephius softened, and spread itself into the fresh skin of the philosopher himself?'[72]

The reporter, suspending his disbelief, accepts an invitation to enter the cave of the 'phantom'. Here he finds retorts and crucibles containing 'secret and many-coloured essences of man and earth', whose merest particle of dust, he is informed, could be made to speak in a way sufficient to hang a murderer: 'But how', he asks, 'can the dust speak?'

> 'Stand by', said Artephius, 'while I question it, and let your eyes attend, for the questioner of nature admits answers only by a way of speech more vivid than that by the ear; speech must be to the eye only, and will here use words that remain with ever-present testimony bearing witness to all people and all times. We trust not passing sounds, gone when they are uttered, present only to those who were present, and dependent for their preservation upon memory that may fail of its trust. The language in which Nature speaks to those who question her is vividly distinct'.[73]

Having thus introduced the language of alchemical demonstration, the next several pages develop an extended series of scenes that connect this animistic imagery with what are clearly recognizable methods of modern toxicological detection. The tour begins with the reduction test, depicted as an 'ordeal' through which 'the glitter of the metal arsenic' emerges out of red heat.[74] Next comes the process of 'the Magus Hugo Reinsch, who spreads a filmy web of copper in which to entangle and catch even the ghost of such a secret'. Artephius invites his visitor to marvel at 'the spell of a Marsh spirit':

> Behold within this crystal prison-house the battle fought between the acid last used and the offended metal zinc; see how they boil with anger as they fight, and the good fairy hydrogen escapes from the uproar. If I place in her way as she is flying anything that contains arsenic, she cannot keep herself from its defilement – she becomes arseniuretted.

The defiled fairy then flies through a 'crystal gallery', depositing some of her arsenic along the way as she eventually plunges into a 'silver sea' where 'the rest of the poison she brings with her darkens also the silver with the hue of crime'.[75] The 'great alchemist of the past and of the present' tests for more than arsenic, employing a 'potash imp' to catch strychnine: 'see how cleverly he telegraphs to me what he has learnt. First he speaks by displaying a deep rich blue signal, which he changes then to purple, then to crimson, then to a brick-red, which last he will continue to display for hours. These words to the eye are unmistakable'.[76]

The mystery enshrouding this journey into the world of alchemical toxicology begins to dissipate at the end of the article. Ascended from the cave and back in his study, the awe-struck traveller begins to reflect on the figure he encountered, recalling his plain, modern dress and mode of speech. He then decides that he had not been transported to some distant place and time. Here he poses a crucial rhetorical question: 'Was the wonder of these things less', he asks, 'than if I had seen them among the owls who frequent the ruins of another Babylon, . . . if these be but modern marvels, and this story of a visit to the Cave of Artephius is discovered to be, after all, only a bookworm's account of an hour with DR. A. S. TAYLOR in the laboratory of GUY'S HOSPITAL?'[77]

How do we answer this question? Is this an account of toxicology as a modern version of alchemical fantasy, or as a credible translation of ancient fantasy into modern scientific reality? Would a more prosaic encounter with 'the modern toxicologist' capture the attention of a readership so well- (even over-) exposed to the vagaries of poison hunting in the early 1860s? Like the subject matter of the story itself, answers are ambiguous. Certainly, the association of Taylor with alchemy suggests the possibility that, like alchemists of old, his discoveries are little more than artefacts of his own ill-disciplined imagination. But Dickens is equally describing a trustworthy, functioning analytical science. The core elements of Artephius's proof – a visual speech, vivid and distinct, and bearing witness to all people and times – constitutes a version of toxicological clarity that, as we have seen, was actively sought after in the laboratory and the courtroom. The tests themselves are depicted with sufficient technical realism to make their functionality recognizable as matters of science. Objections to their possible fallacies, moreover, are built into the story and resolved with a facility that the modern poison hunter would envy. Underdetermination is contained by recourse to concurrent testimony: 'They who sit in the light of nature questioning what is in man', Artephius explains, 'have many servants, and are taught by many voices. One witness may suffice, yet we depend not upon one alone'.[78] Artephius avoids fallacies stemming from impure reagents with equal assurance, refraining from catching his 'ghosts' until after he has 'questioned' his testing material and heard it 'repl[y] that it was itself entirely free from arsenic'.[79] Artephius's parting words resonate against the countless declarations of toxicological promise uttered in previous decades: although the work of detection was by no means simple, 'whenever men are wise enough to make prompt search into the truth, there is no cunning that shall master ours, neither can any poisoner be wise enough to know with certainty how he shall prevent the grave itself from yielding up his secret, or the dead from being raised up by magic of a cave like this into the damning witness of his crime before the face of all the living'.[80]

It is this tension between the recognizable and the strange that makes this encounter with the modern alchemist so interesting. Placing Taylor in a mythic frame enables Dickens to paint a far more univocal and authoritative picture of modern toxicology than Taylor himself could possibly have done. In these pages, toxicology's true, but frustrated, desire can be fulfilled. Dickens's tale in this sense serves at once as a re-articulation and a displacement of modern toxicology's constitutive elements. Poison's capacity to stimulate the public imagination was the source of the toxicologist's pre-eminence as a representative of Victorian medicolegal expertise. Yet this same public imagination required disciplining in order for toxicology to function as an emblematic instance of modern scientific expertise. As a science, toxicology traded on its capacity to produce tangible traces of things unseen. The significance accorded to these traces in turn depended on grounding a set of agreed equivalences (this metal film is the arsenic that caused the death, for example) produced in one place and displayed in another. Both its production and its display, moreover, simultaneously required imagination and were endangered by it. The toxicologist in his laboratory orchestrated plain fact through his complex manipulation, while guarding against enthusiasts and incipient monomaniacs. The courtroom saw poison that was not there, sometimes legitimately (in the toxicologist's tube), sometimes in error (in false stains, or blackened bodies). Dickens's encounter with Taylor, in short, at once captures the reality of a toxicology poised at the cusp of science and the imagination and, by transposing its terrain from fact to fiction, confirms it as a credible enterprise.

We could end here, and might well have done so, but for the serendipity of *All the year round*'s production cycle. 'The Modern alchemist' was the final article to appear in 1862. On the first page of its inaugural 1863 number lay an instalment of *No name*, a serialized novel written by Dickens's protégé, Wilkie Collins. The plot elements of *No name* are fully in keeping with its author's reputation as the leading exponent of the emergent genre of sensation fiction: mistaken and fraudulent identity, marital secrets masked by surface propriety, and poison. Although poison plays but a minor role in *No name*, the story's textual proximity to Dickens's alchemist affords an opportunity to indicate, however briefly, where the story we have followed might be expected to go next. It is with Collins that the continuing complex interplay of poison and the imagination is most strikingly evoked.

Note, first, the chronological and thematic proximity of the sensation novel to the trial of Thomas Smethurst. According to contemporary and modern critics, the sensation genre burst on to the literary scene with the 1859–60 serialization of Collins's *Woman in white*. The core elements of sensation were fully catered for by the details of Smethust's case – a point not lost on commentators of the day. In its initial editorial on the case, *The Times* introduced its readers in a style that would have served well as advertising copy for a Collins novel: 'Who can hope to penetrate into the mysteries of this great town? Who can tell what is passing in any one of the dull uniform rows of houses of which London is made up? . . . Could the secrets of all hearts be opened, could the hidden deeds of all be known, we should be surprised indeed at the taste of the society in the midst of which we are living.'[81]

That poison and sensation were well matched for narrative purposes was a point recognized by literary commentators. In his canonical analysis of the genre, Henry Mansel held that the key to the sensation novel's capacity to thrill was its manipulation of the semblance of modern middle-class normality, the idea that the ordinary and the mundane might belie a more disturbing reality. He illustrates this point with a telling example:

We read with little emotion, though it comes in the form of history, Livy's narrative of the secret poisonings carried on by nearly two hundred Roman ladies; we feel but a feeble interest in the authentic record of the crimes of a Borgia or a Brinvilliers; but we are thrilled with horror, even in fiction, by the thought that such things may be going on around us and among us. The man who shook our hand with a hearty English grasp half an hour ago – the woman whose beauty and grace were the charm of last night, and whose gentle words sent us home better pleased with the world and with ourselves – how exciting to think that under these pleasing outsides may be concealed some demon in human shape, a Count Fosco or a Lady Audley![82]

Throughout his career as a novelist, Collins capitalized on poison's complex cultural resonances to further the cause of sensation.[83] The principal malefactor in *The woman in white*, which is not only considered the first sensation novel but also one of the earliest detective novels, is the Italian nobleman and gentleman chemist Count Fosco, who remarks on the facility of subtle poisoning, and hatches a wild (although unexecuted) poison plot to accomplish his malevolent ends. In his subsequent novels, Collins treats his readers to labyrinthine poison plots involving, among others, Styrian peasants (*Lady and the law*, 1875); poisoning for insurance money (*Haunted hotel*, 1879); re-discovered Borgia poisons (*Jezebel's daughter*, 1880); and poisoning with fraudulently acquired medicines (*Legacy of Cain*, 1889).

But it is in his 1866 novel, *Armadale*, that Collins gives fullest vent to the potential of poisoning as the motor for a sensational plot. The plot centres on doubled, forged identities, through which two men named Allan Armadale are placed in fateful proximity. The key agent in this deception, and the character most involved with manipulating it to her own ends, is the poisoner, Lydia Gwilt. We are introduced to Gwilt by a tale from her childhood, when, as a servant, she forges a letter that facilitates the imposture of one Armadale for the other – a deception, moreover, enabled by the use of poison as a means of inducing temporary incapacitation. In adult life, among her many misdeeds, she becomes associated with a network of gamblers and swindlers, marrying one only to later poison him. Convicted of the crime, she is pardoned by the Home Secretary after a wave of popular protest, and thus allowed to continue to drive the labyrinthine plot forward to its poisonous climax.

Armadale shows Collins putting the narrative power of poison to numerous uses, of which two are most salient here. First, like Dickens's rendering of toxicological alchemy, Collins's text at times seems at pains to defend toxicology against its contemporary critics, as when he comments on the public reception of Gwilt's conviction:

On the evening of the trial, two or three of the young buccaneers of literature went down to two or three newspaper offices, and wrote two or three
heart-rending leading articles on the subject of the proceedings in court.
The next morning the public caught light like tinder; and the prisoner was
tried over again, before an amateur court of justice, in the columns of the
newspapers. All the people who had no personal experience whatever on
the subject seized their pens, and rushed (by kind permission of the editor)
into print. Doctors who had *not* attended the sick man, and who had *not*
been present at the examination of the body, declared by dozens that he had
died a natural death. Barristers without business, who had *not* heard the
evidence, attacked the jury who had heard it, and judged the judge, who had
sat on the bench before some of them were born. The general public followed the lead of the barristers and the doctors, and the young buccaneers
who had set the thing going. Here was the law that they all paid to protect
them actually doing its duty in dreadful earnest! Shocking! shocking! The
British Public rose to protest as one man against the working of its own
machinery.[84]

The passage's savage mockery was a stark and unambiguous reprise of the
circumstances surrounding the Smethurst reprieve. A conviction justly
reached had been subverted by a combination of journalistic oppor-
tunism and second-hand scientific speculation. The science of poison
detection, then, was endangered by the other uses to which a good poison
case could be put. Collins's indignant critique, to be sure, contains its own
tensions, starting with the obvious point that for his critics he was himself the archetypal literary 'buccaneer'. Yet it is important to notice the
prosaic uses of this passage as well – as a transposed, but not much trans-
formed, expiation of an embattled toxicology. Unresolved as a matter of
expert practice, a resituated poison proof might enjoy greater success.

But, of course, Collins's interest in poison was not confined to the
cause of toxicological rehabilitation. As noted above, his plots rehearse
elements of toxicology's agonistic relationship to its object – the presence
in his texts of Styrian peasants, recovered slow poisons and the like, testifying to the unfinished work of disciplining poison. *Armadale's* closing
scenes represent the apogee of this other tendency, neither of directly
supporting nor criticizing, but of unravelling, toxicology's epic struggles
with poison. They involve Gwilt's final treacherous deed when, after
having married one of the Alan Armadales, she conspires to poison the
other in order to achieve her ultimate aim of usurping the eponymous
family's fortune. In this she enlists the unscrupulous Dr Downward, the
epitome of malevolent medical duplicity, who is happy to oblige. Notic-
ing Gwilt's fixation on commonly recognizable poisons, Downward

steers her from the path of literalism, advising her to consider the uses of his innocent-looking medicines:

'My dear lady, what interest can you possibly have in looking at a medical bottle, simply because it happens to be a bottle of poison?' . . . 'I have the interest of looking at it', she said, 'and of thinking, if it got into some people's hands, of the terrible things it might do'. The doctor glanced at his assistant with a compassionate smile. 'Curious, Benjamin', he said, 'the romantic view taken of these drugs of ours by the unscientific mind! My dear lady', he added, turning to Miss Gwilt, 'if *that* is the interest you attach to looking at poisons, you needn't ask me to unlock my cabinet – you need only look about you round the shelves of this room. There are all sorts of medical liquids and substances in those bottles – most innocent, most useful in themselves – which, in combination with other substances and other liquids, become poisons as terrible and as deadly as any that I have in my cabinet under lock and key'.[85]

Downward draws Gwilt's attention to a bottle containing a 'harmless and useful medicine' which he calls 'our Stout Friend'. This 'friend', he declared, 'has made no romantic appearances in courts of law; he has excited no breathless interest in novels; he has played no terrifying part on the stage. There he is, an innocent, inoffensive creature, who troubles nobody with the responsibility of locking him up!' But, in conjunction with another equally accessible substance, and under the proper conditions (which Downward proceeds to detail), the 'friend' will 'kill Sampson himself,

'will kill him in half an hour! Will kill him slowly, without his seeing anything, without his smelling anything, without his feeling anything but sleepiness. Will kill him, and tell the whole College of Surgeons nothing, if they examine him after death, but that he died of apoplexy or congestion of the lungs! What do you think of *that*, my dear lady, in the way of mystery and romance! Is our harmless Stout Friend as interesting *now* as if he rejoiced in the terrible popular fame of the Arsenic and the Strychnine which I keep locked up there?'[86]

With these words, Downward simultaneously extinguishes and sets free the poisoned imagination. Poison had kept the public in its thrall by being figured as an entity at once physically distinct (and thus capable of detection and containment) and evanescent (and thus the stuff of 'mystery and romance'). But so too had toxicology, for it was precisely the 'popular fame' of substances like arsenic and strychnine that under-pinned its standing as the medico-legal bulwark of social order. As

Collins's observation implies, toxicology's own investment in this conception of poison made it complicit in a set of delusions, conjuring fantasies of mastery and contributing to the impotence of its detective efforts. Downward's locked cabinet, in exposing containment as essentially an exercise in displacement, is emblematic of the more general implosion of Victorian toxicology's project of taming, defining, and disciplining. In a world in which anything might be a poison, the work of the poison hunter looks quixotic at best, futile at worst.

Notes

1 *The Times* (28 May 1856), p. 9. The *Examiner* thought the whole proceedings did 'honour to the administration of justice' (31 May 1856), p. 337, while the *Saturday review*, expressing the 'strongest satisfaction' with the entire case, ventured that no other country 'could show so excellent a specimen of perfect logic and freedom from all prejudice as this case has afforded', *Saturday review* 2 (1856), p. 102. For a modern appreciation of the handling of the complex facts of this case by both the prosecution and defence, see David Cairns, *Advocacy and the making of the adversarial criminal trial, 1800–1865* (Oxford: Clarendon Press, 1998), p. 163.

2 'The great trial', *The law times* 27 (1856), p. 110.

3 'The medical evidence in the case of the Queen versus Palmer', *Lancet* 1 (1856), p. 594; 'The trial of William Palmer', *Association medical journal* 4 (n.s.) (1856), p. 455.

4 *The Times* (11 June 1856), p. 5.

5 'Palmer's end', *Examiner* (21 June 1856), p. 386.

6 'Science in the witness-box', *Examiner* (31 May 1856), p. 35.

7 *Ibid.* In this revised interpretative scenario, even the non-expert might have a place: 'The corpse of Cook bore its testimony against the murderer, and Stevens, the kind father-in-law, was struck by its appearance, as he tenderly gazed at it in the coffin'. Other newspapers agreed that the medico-legal evidence against Palmer was collective, with physiology and pathology more important than chemistry. See e.g. *The Times* (5 June 1856), p. 8; *Lloyd's weekly London newspaper* (4 June 1856), p. 6.

8 According to Home Office files, Rees billed for £115; Taylor's bill is not preserved. PRO HO 45/6260/27.

9 'Palmer's end', *Examiner* (21 June 1856), p. 386.

10 'A medical opinion', *Lloyd's* (4 June 1856), p. 6.

11 'Charges of manslaughter against a surgeon', *Lancet* 1 (1856), pp. 692–3.

12 'The medical evidence in the case of the Queen versus Palmer', *Ibid.*, p. 593.

13 *Ibid.*, p. 594.

14 'The scientific evidence on the trial of William Palmer', *Ibid.*, pp. 662–8, p. 667.

15 'The Rugeley poisoning case', *Association medical journal* 4 (n.s.) (1856), pp. 503–4, p. 504. It is noteworthy that the *AMJ*, the forerunner of the *BMJ* and a leading voice of medical professionalization, chose to ignore the more obvious breach of professional ideals – that of a registered practitioner poisoning his patients.

16 'The Rugeley poisoning case', *Association medical journal* 4 (n.s.) (1856), pp. 483–4, p. 483.

17 Alfred Swaine Taylor, 'On poisoning by strychnia, with comments on the medical evidence given at the trial of William Palmer', *Guy's Hospital reports* 2 (3rd ser.) (1856), pp. 269–404. The article was published as a pamphlet by Longman, Brown, Green, Longmans, & Roberts later in the same year.

18 *Ibid.*, pp. 270–1. Emphasis original.

19 *Ibid.*, p. 272.

20 *Ibid.*, p. 271.

21 *Ibid.*, p. 329.

22 *Ibid.*, p. 341.

23 Alfred Swaine Taylor, *On poisons in relation to medical jurisprudence*, 2nd edn (London: John Churchill, 1859), pp. 797–8. Taylor pointedly closes this observation with two page references intended to serve as examples of this tendency – one each to 'mistakes' by the over-enthusiastic Herapath and Letheby.

24 *Ibid.*, p. 213.

25 Alfred Swaine Taylor, *On poisons in relation to medical jurisprudence* (London: John Churchill, 1848), p. 129.

26 *Ibid.* (1859), p. 180.

27 *Ibid.*, p. 182.

28 In his much-expanded 1859 section on strychnine detection (eight times the length of the 1848 version), Taylor goes into detail about the possible sources of fallacy, naming numerous substances which produce colour reactions resembling strychnine, and criticizing 'enthusiastic chemists' who nevertheless rely on colour alone: 'On the whole, in medico-legal practice, it would be unsafe to rely upon colour thus produced in organic extracts, unless we have the corroboration derived from crystalline form and a bitter taste. In the absence of the latter, whatever results the colour test may give, there can be no certainty that strychnia is present'. (*Ibid.*, p. 786).

29 *Ibid.*, p. 206.

30 For example, while Taylor's 1859 review of the existing studies on strychnine absorption was explicitly linked to the Palmer case by Taylor's inclusion of his own 'On poisoning by strychnia' (referred to as containing experimental results 'which formed the basis of the evidence for the prosecution and defence in the case of *Reg. v. Palmer*') the 1875 edition erased any such overt association. The *Guy's* report ('On poisoning') was referenced without mention of either its author (Taylor) or its primary referent (the Palmer case): it

was simply one of a number of recent studies supportive of the proposition that strychnine's properties made detection problematic. Palmer was erased in name – present only implicitly as a chronological trace accounting for the preponderance of studies written in 1856 and 1857 that were included in Taylor's review of the literature. Taylor, *On poisons* (1859), p. 70; *Ibid.* (1875), p. 36.

31 Medical journals were quick to point out that Smethurst's name could not be found in the English, Scottish, or Irish medical directories.

32 *The Times* (5 May 1859), p. 8; (12 May 1859), p. 12.

33 *Ibid.* (21 May 1859), p. 12.

34 *Ibid.*

35 Leonard A. Parry, *Trial of Dr. Smethurst* (Edinburgh and London: William Hodge and Co., 1931), p. 90.

36 Alfred Swaine Taylor, 'Facts and fallacies connected with the research for arsenic and antimony', *Guy's Hospital reports* 6 (3rd ser.) (1860), pp. 201–65, p. 270. Taylor supported this claim by the absence of arsenical contamination of pure copper in the works of Europe's leading chemists: 'In fact, whether among English or French or German writers on chemistry and toxicology', Taylor concluded, 'there is not one who has ever pointed out, or even suspected, that this process would lead to error by reason of the universal presence of arsenic in copper'. *Ibid.*, p. 224.

37 Parry, *Trial of Dr. Smethurst*, p. 95.

38 The judge, Justice Pollock, claimed to have received over 250 letters, petitions and memorials. PRO HO 12/122/37649/93. This file contains scores of similar documents sent directly to the Home Office.

39 'The trial of Thomas Smethurst', *British medical journal* (1859), pp. 725–6, p. 725.

40 'Hanging in doubt', *Lloyd's* (28 August 1859). It was in part as an exercise in purification that three of the defence witnesses wrote to the Home Secretary whilst the verdict was under appeal: given Taylor's use of contaminated copper, they took it as 'a *sacred* duty incumbent on us to entirely repudiate an analysis made with such *impure* materials'. Taylor's practical violation had lead to a blurring of cognitive categories: 'The analysis may be true, it may be false, it may be a mixture of truth and falsity', they lamented – a situation which could only be relieved by months, if not years, of diligent research. *A letter to the Right Honourable Sir George Lewis, ... from three of the medical witnesses for the defence, in the case of Thomas Smethurst* (London: H. Baillière, 1859), p. 30. Emphasis added.

41 'Trial and conviction of Smethurst', *Lancet* 2 (1859), pp. 219–20, p. 220; 'The trial of Thomas Smethurst', *BMJ* (27 August 1859), pp. 702–3, p. 703.

42 Not all welcomed the decision, with the *Saturday review* lamenting, for example, 'that what is called public opinion should be allowed to have the very slightest weight in a case of this kind is one of the greatest calamities that

could befall us. The object of criminal justice', it concluded, 'is not to gratify the passing inclinations of the majority, but to carry out certain rules'. 'The reprieve of Smethurst', *Saturday review* 8 (1859), pp. 304–5, p. 304.

43 The Home Office decided on a full pardon in November 1859. Home Office files show that the decision was reached after lengthy discussions involving criticism not only of Taylor but also of Pollock, who, as the Home Secretary himself observed, 'may have shown too much of the spirit of an advocate and too little of judicial calmness. Probably he had the image of Campbell, in Palmer's case, before his eyes'. However, the Home Secretary, Sir George Cornewall Lewis, insisted on the need to avoid 'the appearance of casting a slur upon Pollock', and on this basis suggested that the public explanation of reprieve should focus not on legal errors but medical ones: 'it might be stated that the decision was made in consequence of new light thrown upon the cause of death by medical opinions obtained since the trial, and called forth by the publicity given to the evidence . . . He ought in fact to see that it has had the effect of extricating him from an immense scrape'. PRO HO 12/122/37649/86, letters from Sir George Cornewall Lewis, 23 August and 6 September 1859.

44 'Smethurst's case: law and medicine', *Lancet* 2 (1859), pp. 542–3, p. 542.

45 *Chemical news* 1 (1859–60), 286.

46 *The Times* (22 August 1859), p. 6.

47 Taylor, 'Facts and fallacies', *Guy's Hospital reports* (1860), pp. 201–65.

48 *Ibid.*, pp. 235–6.

49 *Ibid.*, pp. 237–8.

50 *Ibid.*, p. 238.

51 'The trial of Thomas Smethurst', *BMJ* (3 September 1859), pp. 725–6, p. 725.

52 *Lancet* 2 (1865), pp. 457–9, p. 458.

53 W. S. Austin, 'Secret poisoning', *Temple bar* 6 (1862), pp. 579–84, p. 580. In this article Taylor was subjected to further humiliation: not only was he denied the position of being the source of expert evidence, he was turned into subject matter for another form of evidence – an amateur phrenology ostensibly indulged by Austin: 'seeing him at the Central Criminal Court for the first time, I observed that, while his eye has the brightness and restlessness of a man of genius, and the bumps that (phrenologically speaking) denoted keenness of observation and rapidity in acquisition, exactly the reverse is the case with those which are supposed to be the seat of the reflective and reasoning faculties'. *Ibid.*

54 *The Times* (12 December 1868), p. 9.

55 Robert Christison, 'On the present state of medidcal evidence', *Edinburgh medical review* 23 (n.s.) (1851), p. 401–30, p. 403.

56 *The Times* (5 September 1859), p. 8.

57 This debate is discussed in Christopher Hamlin, 'Scientific method and expert witnessing', *Social studies of science* 76 (1986), pp. 485–513, and more

fully in Tal Golan, *Laws of men and laws of nature: the history of scientific expert testimony in England and America* (Cambridge MA and London: Havard University Press, 2004), ch. 3.

58 *BMJ* (1859), pp. 725–6, p. 725.

59 *Lancet* 2 (1859), p. 650. I explore the tensions between the desire for officially sanctioned expertise and the appeal of native institutions guaranteeing English liberties, in Ian Burney, *Bodies of evidence: medicine and the politics of the English inquest, 1830–1926* (Baltimore and London: Johns Hopkins University Press, 2000). For an analysis of the historical roots of the differing place of English and continental medico-legal experts, see Catherine Crawford, 'Legalizing medicine: early modern legal systems and the growth of medico-legal knowledge', in Michael Clark and Catherine Crawford (eds), *Legal medicine in history* (Cambridge: Cambridge University Press, 1994), and, more fully, Crawford, 'The emergence of medical jurisprudence: Medical evidence in English courts, 1750–1850', Ph.D. dissertation, University of Oxford, 1987.

60 'Proposed toxicological commission', *Chemical news* 1 (1859–60), p. 49. Emphasis original.

61 Robert Angus Smith, 'Science in our courts of law', *Journal of the Society of Arts* 7 (1860), pp. 135–42, p. 137.

62 Hamlin, 'Scientific method and expert witnessing', especially pp. 494–5. See also Tal Golan, 'The history of scientific expert testimony in the English courtroom', *Science in context* 12:1 (1999), pp. 7–32, esp. pp. 20–5. Both Hamlin and Golan cite Frank Turner's work for a broader framework for their analyses, especially F. Turner, 'Public science in Britain, 1880–1919', *Isis* 71 (1980), pp. 589–608.

63 There were, to be sure, partial successes, most notably the appointment of official Home Office analysts in 1871, experts who could be called on by the state in cases of special difficulty. These analysts retained at least nominal independence, however, in that they were nominated by the Royal Colleges, and were in principle free to appear for the defence as well as the prosecution. For more, see Jennifer Ward, 'Origins and development of forensic medicine and forensic science in England, 1823–1946', Ph.D. dissertation, Open University, 1993, ch. 4.

64 The scientific cases against Palmer and Smethurst, recall, both involved two analysts – an arrangement that had guaranteed neither success nor expert solidarity. In the wake of Smethurst, for example, Odling publicly denounced his laboratory collaborator, denying what he took to be Taylor's efforts to distribute blame: 'he has indulged largely in misrepresentation, not merely by suppressing some points and modifying others, but also by attributing to me, in more or less distinct terms, processes which I never performed, and opinions which I never entertained'. *Pharmaceutical journal* 2 (2nd ser.) (1860–61), p. 212.

65 'The detection and determination of arsenic', *Lancet* 1 (1901), p. 1700.

66 James Fitzjames Stephen, 'On trial by jury, and the evidence of experts', *Papers read before the Juridical Society* 2 (1858–63) (London: W. Maxwell, 1863), pp. 236–49, p. 238. Stephen returned to this theme in his later writings, using the cases of Palmer and Smethurst to illustrate his points. See J. F. Stephen, *History of the criminal law in England*, 3 vols, (London: Macmillan, 1883), 3, pp. 423–5, pp. 464–5.

67 Stephen, 'On trial by jury', pp. 243–4. Stephen's suspicion of the applicability of highly refined science to the conduct of public justice points to a larger problem about looking to technical sophistication to resolve contention. As we saw in the early response to the 'nicety' of results afforded by the Marsh test, a process's very refinement might itself become the focus of controversy. Contemporaries acknowledged toxicology's susceptibility to what modern sociologists of science would call 'experimental regress'. Tests for the detection of poison, the *Lancet* wrote in 1910, 'become constantly more detailed and more conclusive. The elaborate nature of the tests used, however, and even the precision claimed for the deductions made from their results, not unnaturally supply material for the advocate which it is his duty to make use of when criticising evidence vitally affecting his client. If a process is of so subtle a nature, he reasons to the jury, may not a fundamental error as to the deductions to be drawn from observed facts, or in the application of a test, affect the result when a minute quantity of a poison is alleged to be present in a small portion of a human body, and may not that error vitiate the whole proceeding'? 'Arsenic and murder by poisoning', *Lancet* 1 (1912), pp. 1070–1, p. 1070.

68 Stephen, 'On trial by jury', 249.

69 'The modern Crichtons', *Blackwood's Edinburgh magazine* 96 (1864), pp. 282–6, p. 284, cited in *Chemical news* 6 (1864–65), p. 318.

70 'Strychnine', *Household words* 13 (1 May 1856), pp. 420–4; 'The demeanour of murderers', *Ibid.* (14 June 1856), pp. 505–7.

71 'Five new points of criminal law', *All the year round* 1 (24 September 1859), p. 517.

72 'The modern alchemist', *Ibid.* 8 (1862–63), pp. 380–4, p. 380.

73 *Ibid.*, p. 382.

74 *Ibid.*

75 *Ibid.*, p. 383.

76 *Ibid.*, pp. 383–4.

77 *Ibid.*, p. 384.

78 *Ibid.*, p. 382.

79 *Ibid.*, p. 383.

80 *Ibid.*, p. 384.

81 *The Times* (22 August 1859), p. 6.

82 'Sensation novels', *Quarterly review* 113 (1863), pp. 481–514, p. 489. There is

an extensive literature on the rise of the sensation novel, including Winifred Hughes, *The maniac in the cellar: sensation novels of the 1860s* (Princeton: Princeton University Press, 1980); Jenny Bourne Taylor, *In the secret theatre of home: Wilkie Collins, sensation narrative, and nineteenth-century psychology* (London and New York: Routledge, 1988); and John Sutherland, 'Wilkie Collins and the origins of the sensation novel', *Dickens studies annual* 20 (1991), pp. 243–57.

83   Note also Collins's journalistic interest in poison: he worked as a reporter for the *Leader* at the time of the Palmer case, with Thomas Boyle claiming that he had in fact served as its Rugeley correspondent. It was his experience with the Palmer trial, John Sutherland argues, that inspired him to write *Woman in white* as a vindication of circumstantial evidence. Thomas Boyle, *Black swine in the sewers of Hampstead: beneath the surface of Victorian sensationalism* (London: Penguin, 1989), ch. 9; Sutherland, 'Wilkie Collins and the origins'. See also Kirk H. Beetz, 'Wilkie Collins and the *Leader*', *Victorian periodicals review* 15:1 (1982), pp. 20–9.

84   Wilkie Collins, *Armadale* (London: Penguin Books, 1995), p. 530. Emphasis original.

85   *Ibid.*, p. 641. Emphasis original.

86   *Ibid.*, p. 642. Emphasis original. I am grateful to my colleague Vladimir Jankovic for several fruitful discussions about the implications of Downward's revelation.

Index

Note: numbers in *italics* refer to illustrations; n indicates a note

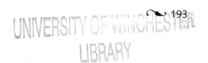

Lightning Source UK Ltd.
Milton Keynes UK
UKOW04f1318291117
313566UK00001B/66/P